T ◆ H ◆ E
1200-Calorie-a-Day
Menu Cookbook

T◆H◆E
1200-Calorie-a-Day Menu Cookbook

Quick and Easy Recipes for
Delicious Low-Fat Breakfasts, Lunches,
Dinners, and Desserts

NANCY S. HUGHES

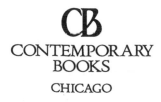

CONTEMPORARY
BOOKS
CHICAGO

Library of Congress Cataloging-in-Publication Data

Hughes, Nancy S.
    The 1200-calorie-a-day menu cookbook : quick and easy recipes for delicious low-fat breakfasts, lunches, dinners, and desserts / Nancy S. Hughes.
       p.   cm.
    Includes index.
    ISBN 0-8092-3633-8
    1. Reducing diets—Recipes.   2. Low-fat diet—Recipes.   I. Title.
II. Title: Twelve hundred-calorie-a-day menu cookbook.
RM222.2.H847   1994
641.5′635—dc20   94-26729
                                         CIP

Featured on the front cover: French Toast with Warm Maple Syrup and Fresh Bananas, Sausage Links, and Cold Milk; Mediterranean Couscous Salad with Fresh Limes, Cucumbers, and Tomatoes; Sliced Turkey with Fresh Mushroom Gravy, Whipped Potatoes, Peppered Peas, and Apricot Halves; and Ladyfinger Strawberry Spokes.

Cover design by Georgene Sainati
Cover photograph by Rick Osentoski, Envision

Published by Contemporary Books, Inc.
Two Prudential Plaza, Chicago, Illinois 60601-6790
Manufactured in the United States of America
International Standard Book Number: 0-8092-3633-8
10   9   8   7   6   5   4   3   2   1

This book is lovingly dedicated
to my husband,
Greg,
for the steadfast guidance and
unconditional love, especially through
the cooking marathons . . .

and to my children,
My son Will, 18—for his tolerant endurance
and independence in creating his own
culinary favorites.

My daughter Anne, 15—for her willingness to
taste every experiment at a moment's notice
and her subtle sense of humor.

My son Taft, 10—for his overwhelming
eagerness to learn and his ability to adjust
to every situation presented.

CONTENTS

❧

❧

ACKNOWLEDGMENTS

Special thanks to:

My in-laws, for the seemingly never-ending conversations on calories and fat grams over the dinner table,

Eunice Swift, whose love and knowledge of food are endless,

Mrs. Rose Guibault, for a very favorite family recipe,

My friends, for being understanding while I was locked in my kitchen,

and, especially,

My dad, whose attitude toward life and work has inspired me beyond words.

INTRODUCTION

This book contains low-fat, low-calorie recipes for breakfasts, lunches, dinners, and desserts—
never to exceed 1,200 calories for the entire day. All breakfasts and lunches are 350 calories
each, all dinners are 400 calories, and all desserts are 100 calories. No matter which meals
are chosen, the total will always add up to 1,200 calories for the day!

Today there is a strong emphasis on the importance of good eating habits. Preparing low-
fat, low-calorie meals, trying to *maintain* a low daily calorie count and control fat intake can
be a true challenge—just the thing we all need to add to our already overloaded lives. Taking
time to figure exactly how many calories and fat grams are being consumed can be
troublesome and frustrating. This, in turn, may lead to giving up on the notion that delicious
low-fat, low-calorie meals can be part of your everyday diet. Therefore, I've written this book
to provide low-calorie meals that are low in fat for the entire day *every* day.

Eating healthy *is* very important, but many feel that doing so means forsaking those
familiar favorites, such as ham and eggs, rich sauces, and cheese-smothered dishes. Unfor-
tunately, we need familiar foods to provide comfort, relief from stress, stability, and enjoyment
on a fairly regular basis. Otherwise "roller coaster" dieting is inevitable.

In this book, I've provided a variety of meals ranging from home-style favorites to the latest
trends. Choose from weekday and weekend breakfasts, lunches for home or the workplace,
hearty dinners, and, of course, those ever-needed desserts. I've included a variety of dishes
utilizing all of the major food groups to keep eating healthy *and* interesting.

As in my previous books, the recipes are easy to prepare, created to please the entire family,
using easily obtainable ingredients. The majority of the meals contain 20 percent or less of
their total calorie content from fat; *all* contain less than 30 percent. These totals are listed at
the beginning of each meal. Many of the main courses for dinner may be used for lunches.
By using a thermos, warming dishes in the microwave, and simply packing salad dressings
separately, you multiply your brown-bagging choices.

This is not a diet plan, but rather a comprehensive collection of recipes that you can use
to help limit your calorie and fat intake and, at the same time, enjoy meals without the guilt

and without the calculator! Whether you're in the mood for something old and familiar or something new and exciting, in a hurry or taking it slow, you don't have to eat "wrong" to feel satisfied anymore.

Besides providing the recipes, I hope this book can be a learning experience. There is a Chinese proverb that says, "Give a man a fish and you have fed him a meal; teach him to fish and you have fed him for life." I hope I can "teach you to fish" so that you know how healthy meals can be a part of your life forever.

Enjoy!

Nancy S. Hughes

T ◆ H ◆ E
1200-Calorie-a-Day
Menu Cookbook

BREAKFASTS

Creamed Eggs on Toast with Fresh Tangerine Slices

Skillet Ham, Over-Easy Eggs, Toast, and Chilled Fresh Orange Juice

Egg and Bacon Stacks with Dijon Cheese Sauce

Early Morning Rush Egg Sandwich, Chilled Fresh Orange Juice,
and Sweet Red Grapes

Ham and Swiss Quiche with Scallions, Toast, and Fresh Strawberries

Mexican Breakfast Rollups and Summer Fruits with Yogurt

Overnight Egg Casserole with Sausage and Cheese, Citrus Cups,
and Chilled Tomato Juice

Diced Potatoes with Sausage and Stewed Apples

French Toast with Warm Maple Syrup and Fresh Bananas,
Sausage Links, and Cold Milk

Sausage and Gravy over Biscuits and Chilled Tomato Juice

Winter Morning Cinnamon Apples, Sausage Links,
and Raisin English Muffins with Cream Cheese

Crispy Mexican Tortilla Sunrise, Fresh Berries, and Tropical Spritzer

Double-Quick Country Drop Biscuits, Scrambled Eggs,
Canadian Bacon, and Grapefruit

Camp-Style Potato Patties with Bacon, Toast, and Fresh Peach Slices

Blueberry Shortcake Cobbler, Canadian Bacon, and Cold Milk

Buttermilk Pancakes with Blueberry Sauce, Canadian Bacon,
and Sliced Fresh Oranges

Cinnamon Shortcakes with Fresh Peaches, Vanilla Cream, and Ham Slices

Panfried Steak and Hash Brown Potatoes

Cheese Grits, Broiled Tomatoes, Warm Bagels, and Fresh Melon

Down-Home Tomato Gravy and Grits, Canadian Bacon,
Toast, and Fresh Melon Slices

Fresh Tomato and Provolone Pizza Quiche

Cherry Crumble and Cinnamon-Vanilla Yogurt

Puffed Blintzes with Rich Cheesecake Sauce and Raspberries
and Mixed Fruit Smoothies

Pecan Caramel Coffee Cake, Fresh Melon, and Cold Milk

Fresh Banana–Oat Bread and Vanilla Yogurt with Sliced Fresh Peaches

Blueberry-Oatmeal Muffins and Sliced Bananas with Vanilla Yogurt

Pecan-Pumpkin Bran Muffins and Fruit with Spiced Orange Cream

Bountiful Fruits and Cereal, Toast, and Chilled Tomato Juice

Citrus-Sweetened Fruit with Apricot-Topped English Muffins

Individual Fruit Platters with Hot Popovers

CREAMED EGGS ON TOAST WITH FRESH TANGERINE SLICES

Serves 4

Total calories per serving: 343
Total fat per serving: 10.9 g (29%)

CREAMED EGGS ON TOAST *(302 calories, 10.7 g fat per serving)*

2 tablespoons light margarine
2½ cups skim milk
3 tablespoons all-purpose flour
1 teaspoon butter-flavored Molly McButter
¼ teaspoon salt
⅛ teaspoon black pepper
8 slices light bread, toasted and halved diagonally
8 large hard-cooked eggs, 2 yolks discarded
Paprika for garnish

1. Place a large nonstick skillet over medium heat; add margarine and melt. In a bowl, whisk together milk, flour, butter flavoring, salt, and pepper until well blended. Increase heat to medium-high and add milk mixture to melted margarine in skillet. Cook, stirring constantly, until thickened. Remove from heat.

2. Arrange four toast halves on each plate. Slice eggs and egg whites. Top each serving with 1½ whole eggs and ½ egg white. Spoon one-fourth of the sauce (about ½ cup) over each serving. Sprinkle with paprika and serve immediately.

FRESH TANGERINE SLICES *(41 calories, 0.2 g fat per serving)*

4 medium-sized tangerines
1 teaspoon powdered sugar

Peel and section tangerines. Place one-fourth of the slices on each of four small serving plates. Sprinkle ¼ teaspoon sugar over each and serve immediately.

SKILLET HAM, OVER-EASY EGGS, TOAST, AND CHILLED FRESH ORANGE JUICE

Serves 4

Total calories per serving: 345
Total fat per serving: 8.6 g (23%)

SKILLET HAM *(72 calories, 2.4 g fat per serving)*

Butter-flavored cooking spray
8 1-ounce slices turkey ham

1. Preheat oven to warm.
2. Coat a large nonstick skillet with cooking spray and place over high heat for 1 minute. Add four slices ham and cook for 2 minutes or until richly browned on bottom. Turn and cook for 1 minute longer. Set on an ovenproof plate and place in warm oven. Repeat with remaining ham and place in warm oven.

OVER-EASY EGGS *(82 calories, 5.8 g fat per serving)*

Butter-flavored cooking spray
4 large eggs
Black pepper to taste

1. Preheat oven to warm.
2. Liberally coat a large nonstick skillet with cooking spray and place over medium heat for 1 minute. Carefully crack 1 egg into skillet, being careful not to break yolk. Cook for 2½ minutes. Turn carefully with a spatula and cook for 1 minute longer. Sprinkle with pepper. Set on a platter and place in warm oven while cooking remaining eggs.

TOAST *(108 calories, 0 g fat per serving)*

8 slices light bread
8 teaspoons all-fruit spread (any flavor)

Toast bread. Top each slice with 1 teaspoon spread and serve.

CHILLED FRESH ORANGE JUICE *(83 calories, 0.4 g fat per serving)*

3 cups fresh-squeezed orange juice, chilled

Serve ¾ cup juice in each of four glasses.

EGG AND BACON STACKS WITH DIJON CHEESE SAUCE

Serves 4

Total calories per serving: 346
Total fat per serving: 10.8 g (28%)

8 ½-ounce slices Oscar Mayer 93 percent fat-free Canadian bacon
4 large eggs
2 cups skim milk
2 tablespoons cornstarch
½ cup (2 ounces) grated reduced-fat sharp cheddar cheese
1 tablespoon plus 1 teaspoon Dijon mustard
2 teaspoons fresh lemon juice
1 teaspoon butter-flavored Molly McButter
¼ teaspoon salt
⅛ teaspoon cayenne pepper
Black pepper to taste
4 English muffins, halved and toasted
Paprika for garnish
Fresh lemon wedges for serving

1. Preheat oven to warm.
2. Set bacon on an ovenproof plate and place in warm oven.
3. Place 1½ inches water in a large skillet. Bring to a boil and reduce heat to low. Crack eggs into skillet, being careful not to break yolks. Simmer for 3–5 minutes, or until egg whites are firm. Using a slotted spoon, transfer eggs to an ovenproof plate and place in warm oven.
4. In a nonstick saucepan, combine milk and cornstarch and stir until cornstarch dissolves. Place over medium heat, stir with a spatula, and cook until thickened. Remove from heat and stir in cheese, mustard, lemon juice, butter flavoring, salt, cayenne, and black pepper.
5. Place two muffin halves on each of four plates and top with two slices bacon and one egg. Pour one-fourth of the sauce over each serving. Sprinkle with paprika and serve immediately with lemon wedges.

EARLY MORNING RUSH EGG SANDWICH, CHILLED FRESH ORANGE JUICE, AND SWEET RED GRAPES

Serves 4

Total calories per serving: 349
Total fat per serving: 5.3 g (14%)

EARLY MORNING RUSH EGG SANDWICH (208 calories, 4.6 g fat per serving)

2 8-ounce cartons egg substitute
⅓ cup evaporated skim milk
½ teaspoon Worcestershire sauce
⅛ teaspoon black pepper or to taste
¼ pound turkey ham, sliced thin and chopped
Cooking spray
8 slices light bread
2 tablespoons plus 2 teaspoons light margarine

1. In a mixing bowl, combine egg substitute, evaporated milk, Worcestershire sauce, and pepper. Whisk until well blended, then stir in turkey ham.
2. Liberally coat a large nonstick skillet with cooking spray and place over medium-high heat for 1 minute. Add egg mixture. When edges become firm, use a spatula to push set egg to center of skillet, allowing uncooked egg to flow to edges. Gently turn until desired consistency.
3. Toast bread and spread 1 teaspoon margarine on each slice. Place one-fourth of the egg mixture on buttered side of four pieces of toast and top with remaining pieces of toast, butter side down. Serve immediately.

CHILLED FRESH ORANGE JUICE (83 calories, 0.4 g fat per serving)

3 cups fresh-squeezed orange juice, chilled

Serve ¾ cup juice in each of four glasses

SWEET RED GRAPES (58 calories, 0.3 g fat per serving)

4 cups seedless red grapes

Rinse grapes and serve in four small serving bowls.

HAM AND SWISS QUICHE WITH SCALLIONS, TOAST, AND FRESH STRAWBERRIES

Serves 4

Total calories per serving: 332
Total fat per serving: 5.7 g (16%)

HAM AND SWISS QUICHE WITH SCALLIONS (179 calories, 5.1 g fat per serving)

Cooking spray
¼ pound turkey ham, sliced thin
  and chopped
1 cup evaporated skim milk
1 tablespoon plus 2 teaspoons
  cornstarch
1 cup skim milk
1 8-ounce carton egg substitute
½ teaspoon dry mustard
⅛ teaspoon black pepper
⅛ teaspoon ground nutmeg
¼ cup chopped scallion
½ cup (2 ounces) grated reduced-
  fat Swiss cheese
½ cup (2-ounces) grated part-
  skim mozzarella cheese
Paprika for garnish

1. Preheat oven to 425°F.
2. Coat a large skillet with cooking spray and place over medium-high heat for 1 minute. Add turkey ham and brown lightly.
3. Meanwhile, in a mixing bowl, combine evaporated milk and cornstarch. Whisk until cornstarch dissolves, then add skim milk, egg substitute, dry mustard, pepper, and nutmeg. Whisk until well blended. Stir in scallion, cheeses, and turkey ham.
4. Coat a 9-inch deep-dish glass pie pan with cooking spray and pour egg mixture into it. Sprinkle with paprika. Bake for 15 minutes. Reduce heat to 300°F and bake for 45 minutes longer or until a knife inserted in center comes out clean. Let stand for 5 minutes before cutting into four wedges and serving.

TOAST (108 calories, 0 g fat per serving)

8 slices light bread
8 teaspoons all-fruit spread
  (any flavor)

Toast bread. Top each slice with 1 teaspoon spread and serve.

FRESH STRAWBERRIES (45 calories, 0.6 g fat per serving)

4 cups strawberries

Rinse and hull strawberries. Slice, if desired, and serve in small bowls

MEXICAN BREAKFAST ROLLUPS AND SUMMER FRUITS WITH YOGURT

Serves 4

Total calories per serving: 330
Total fat per serving: 3.2 g (9%)

MEXICAN BREAKFAST ROLLUPS *(240 calories, 2.9 g fat per serving)*

2 8-ounce cartons egg substitute
⅓ cup evaporated skim milk
1 teaspoon chili powder
½ teaspoon ground cumin
¼ teaspoon cayenne pepper
¼ teaspoon salt
¼ teaspoon black pepper
2 medium-sized tomatoes, seeded and chopped (about 1 cup)
½ cup finely chopped green bell pepper
¼ pound turkey ham, sliced thin and chopped
Cooking spray
1 tablespoon plus 1 teaspoon light margarine
8 6-inch corn tortillas, warmed

1. In a medium-sized mixing bowl, combine egg substitute, milk, chili powder, cumin, cayenne, salt, and black pepper. Whisk together until well blended. Gently stir in tomato, bell pepper, and ham.
2. Coat a large nonstick skillet with cooking spray and place over medium-high heat for 1 minute. Pour egg mixture into skillet and cook, stirring occasionally with a spatula, until eggs are set.
3. Spread ½ teaspoon margarine evenly over each tortilla and place one-eighth of the scrambled egg mixture in center of each buttered tortilla. Fold in edges and place two rollups seam down on each plate and serve immediately.

Variation: Omit salt and green bell pepper and add ½ cup *drained* canned green chilies.

SUMMER FRUITS WITH YOGURT *(90 calories, 0.3 g fat per serving)*

2 cups nonfat yogurt (any flavor)
2 cups strawberry slices
2 medium-sized kiwifruits, peeled and sliced

Place ½ cup yogurt in each of four small serving bowls. Decoratively top each with ½ cup strawberry slices and one-fourth of the kiwifruit slices.

OVERNIGHT EGG CASSEROLE WITH SAUSAGE AND CHEESE, CITRUS CUPS, AND CHILLED TOMATO JUICE

Serves 4

Total calories per serving: 350
Total fat per serving: 9.6 g (25%)

OVERNIGHT EGG CASSEROLE WITH SAUSAGE AND CHEESE
(277 calories, 9.6 g fat per serving)

Cooking spray
½ pound bulk turkey sausage
¼ teaspoon fennel seed
¼ teaspoon dried oregano leaves
¼ pound French bread, cut into
  ½-inch cubes
1 8-ounce carton egg substitute
⅔ cup skim milk
½ cup evaporated skim milk
1 teaspoon dry mustard
⅛–¼ teaspoon cayenne pepper
Dash black pepper
Paprika for garnish
½ cup (2 ounces) grated reduced-
  fat sharp cheddar cheese

1. Coat a nonstick skillet with cooking spray and place over medium-high heat for 1 minute. Add sausage, fennel, and oregano, breaking up sausage with a knife and fork, and cook until brown. Transfer to paper towels and set aside.
2. Coat an 8-inch square baking pan with cooking spray and line bottom with cubed bread. Sprinkle meat over bread. In a mixing bowl, combine egg substitute, skim milk, evaporated milk, dry mustard, cayenne, and black pepper. Pour over sausage and bread and sprinkle with paprika. Cover with foil and refrigerate overnight.
3. Preheat oven to 350°F. Bake covered casserole for 55 minutes. Remove from oven, discard foil, sprinkle with cheese, and let stand for 5 minutes to finish cooking casserole and melt cheese. Cut into four sections and serve.

CITRUS CUPS *(38 calories, 0 g fat per serving)*

1 medium-sized orange, peeled
1 8-ounce can grapefruit sections,
  drained

1. Separate orange sections. Cut each section into thirds.
2. Combine orange and grapefruit sections. Serve one-fourth of the mixture in each of four small serving bowls.

CHILLED TOMATO JUICE *(35 calories, 0 g fat per serving)*

3 cups tomato juice, chilled

Serve ¾ cup juice in each of four glasses.

DICED POTATOES WITH SAUSAGE AND STEWED APPLES

Serves 4

Total calories per serving: 349
Total fat per serving: 8.5 g (22%)

DICED POTATOES WITH SAUSAGE *(285 calories, 8.2 g fat per serving)*

Cooking spray
6 ounces turkey sausage links, cut
   into ⅛-inch rounds
1½ pounds unpeeled red
   potatoes, diced
1 cup chopped yellow onion
1 cup chopped green bell pepper
1 tablespoon plus 1 teaspoon
   chopped fresh parsley
⅛ teaspoon black pepper or to
   taste
⅛ teaspoon cayenne pepper
1 tablespoon extra-virgin olive oil
¼ teaspoon salt

1. Preheat oven to 350°F.
2. Coat a dutch oven (preferably cast iron) with cooking spray, place over medium-high heat, add sausage, and brown. Remove from heat and set aside.
3. Rinse potatoes with cold water, drain well, and dry with paper towels. Combine potatoes with sausage in dutch oven. Add onion, bell pepper, parsley, black pepper, cayenne, and oil. Toss well to coat thoroughly. Cover tightly and bake for 35 minutes or until potatoes are tender. Stir in salt, cover, and let stand for 5 minutes before serving to allow flavors to blend.

STEWED APPLES *(64 calories, 0.3 g fat per serving)*

2 cups water
2 medium-sized Red Delicious
   apples, cored and cut into
   ½-inch wedges
2 tablespoons frozen apple juice
   concentrate
1 teaspoon vanilla extract

In a medium-sized saucepan, bring water to a boil. Add apple wedges, return to a boil, reduce heat, and simmer, uncovered, for 4 minutes or until *just* tender. Remove from heat. Drain well and place in a serving bowl. To saucepan, add apple juice concentrate and vanilla and place over medium-low heat to warm slightly. Pour over apples, cover, and let stand for 2–3 minutes to blend flavors.

FRENCH TOAST WITH WARM MAPLE SYRUP
AND FRESH BANANAS, SAUSAGE LINKS, AND COLD MILK

Serves 4

Total calories per serving: 344
Total fat per serving: 6.8 g (18%)

FRENCH TOAST WITH WARM MAPLE SYRUP AND FRESH BANANAS
(186 calories, 0.4 g fat per serving)

¾ cup skim milk
¼ cup egg substitute
1½ teaspoons vanilla extract *or* ¼
    teaspoon vanilla butter nut
    flavoring
¼ teaspoon ground cinnamon
4 slices light bread
Butter-flavored cooking spray
¼ cup lite maple syrup, heated
1⅓ cups sliced bananas
Ground nutmeg for garnish

1. In a mixing bowl, combine milk, egg substitute, vanilla, and cinnamon; blend thoroughly. Dip bread slices in mixture and let bread absorb it.
2. Liberally coat a large nonstick skillet with cooking spray and place over medium-high heat for 1 minute. Add bread slices and cook for 6 minutes. Turn and cook for 5–7 minutes longer or until golden brown. Place one slice of French toast on each of four plates, spoon 1 tablespoon warm syrup over, and serve ⅓ cup banana slices alongside. Sprinkle bananas with nutmeg and serve immediately.

Variation: Omit maple syrup and use 2 teaspoons powdered sugar mixed with ⅛ teaspoon ground cinnamon per serving.

SAUSAGE LINKS *(90 calories, 6 g fat per serving)*

Cooking spray
10 ounces turkey sausage links,
    cut into fourths

Coat a large nonstick skillet with cooking spray and place over medium-high heat for 1 minute. Split each sausage piece lengthwise, place in skillet, and cook until browned, about 5 minutes, turning occasionally.

COLD MILK *(68 calories, 0.4 g fat per serving)*

3 cups skim milk, chilled

Serve ¾ cup milk in each of four glasses.

SAUSAGE AND GRAVY OVER BISCUITS AND CHILLED TOMATO JUICE

Serves 4

Total calories per serving: 327
Total fat per serving: 6.6 g (18%)

SAUSAGE AND GRAVY OVER BISCUITS *(292 calories, 6.6 g per serving)*

Cooking spray
6 ounces bulk turkey sausage
1¾ cups skim milk
2 tablespoons all-purpose flour
2 teaspoons butter-flavored Molly McButter
¼ teaspoon black pepper
1 7½-ounce can Pillsbury Buttermilk Biscuits

1. Preheat oven to 450°F.
2. Coat a skillet, preferably cast iron, with cooking spray. Place over medium heat, add sausage, and stir and crumble with a fork. Cook until done. In a bowl, whisk together milk, flour, butter flavoring, and pepper until thoroughly blended. Add to cooked sausage in skillet. Stir occasionally using a spatula and cook until thickened, about 8 minutes.
3. Meanwhile, place biscuits on a baking sheet and bake for 5 minutes or until done.
4. At serving time, split eight of the biscuits, saving two for another use, and place four halves on each plate. Spoon one-fourth of the sausage mixture over biscuits and serve immediately.

CHILLED TOMATO JUICE *(35 calories, 0 g fat per serving)*

3 cups tomato juice, chilled

Serve ¾ cup juice in each of four glasses.

WINTER MORNING CINNAMON APPLES, SAUSAGE LINKS, AND RAISIN ENGLISH MUFFINS WITH CREAM CHEESE

Serves 4

Total calories per serving: 349
Total fat per serving: 7.9 g (20%)

WINTER MORNING CINNAMON APPLES (79 calories, 0.4 g fat per serving)

2 large Red Delicious apples, halved and cored
4 teaspoons red-hot cinnamon heart candies
4 teaspoons fresh orange juice or water

1. Preheat oven to 350°F.
2. Slightly crumple a sheet of aluminum foil to line bottom of a 9-inch square baking dish. (This allows apples to sit evenly.) Place apple halves on top. Place 1 teaspoon candies in cavity of each apple. Spoon 1 teaspoon orange juice or water over candies. Bake for 35 minutes or until just tender. Spoon any accumulated juices over tops of apples and serve.

SAUSAGE LINKS (90 calories, 6 g fat per serving)

6 ounces turkey sausage links

1. Preheat broiler.
2. Place links on broiler rack and broil for 3–5 minutes, or until done. Remove from oven. Cut each link into four pieces. Place one-fourth of the links on each of four plates and serve.

RAISIN ENGLISH MUFFINS WITH CREAM CHEESE (180 calories, 1.5 g fat per serving)

4 raisin English muffins
4 tablespoons fat-free cream cheese

Split English muffins and toast each half. Spread 1½ teaspoons cream cheese over each half. Place two muffin halves on each of four plates and serve.

CRISPY MEXICAN TORTILLA SUNRISE, FRESH BERRIES, AND TROPICAL SPRITZER

Serves 4

Total calories per serving: 345
Total fat per serving: 7.5 g (20%)

CRISPY MEXICAN TORTILLA SUNRISE *(185 calories, 7 g fat per serving)*

Cooking spray
5 ounces bulk turkey sausage
4 8-inch corn tortillas
¾ cup (3 ounces) grated part-skim mozzarella cheese
1 4-ounce can green chilies, drained
1 large tomato, seeded and chopped (about 1 cup)
½ teaspoon chili powder
½ teaspoon dried oregano leaves
Black pepper to taste

1. Preheat oven to 475°F.
2. Coat a nonstick skillet with cooking spray and place over medium-high heat for 1 minute. Add sausage, breaking it up with a knife and fork. Cook until done. Drain on paper towels.
3. Place two tortillas on each of two large baking sheets. Sprinkle each with 3 tablespoons grated cheese, 2 tablespoons chilies, ¼ cup chopped tomato, and one-fourth of the sausage. Sprinkle ⅛ teaspoon chili powder and ⅛ teaspoon oregano on top of sausage, then add black pepper. Bake for 4 minutes. Serve immediately.

Note: For a softer tortilla, bake in a 350°F oven just until cheese melts.

FRESH BERRIES *(85 calories, 0.3 g fat per serving)*

2 cups fresh blueberries
4 cups sliced strawberries

Rinse blueberries, discarding any stems remaining on berries. Combine fruits. Place one-fourth of mixture in each of four bowls. Serve.

TROPICAL SPRITZER *(75 calories, 0.2 g fat per serving)*

2 cups pineapple-orange juice
2 tablespoons plus 2 teaspoons frozen grapefruit juice concentrate
½ teaspoon coconut extract
Ice cubes
1 cup sparkling mineral water

In a pitcher, combine pineapple-orange juice, grapefruit juice concentrate, and coconut extract. Chill. At serving time, fill four glasses with ice, add mineral water to juice and stir gently, and pour equal amounts into each glass. Serve immediately.

DOUBLE-QUICK COUNTRY DROP BISCUITS, SCRAMBLED EGGS, CANADIAN BACON, AND GRAPEFRUIT

Serves 4

Total calories per serving: 349
Total fat per serving: 4.2 g (11%)

DOUBLE-QUICK COUNTRY DROP BISCUITS *(184 calories, 2 g fat per serving)*

1¾ cups all-purpose flour
2 tablespoons margarine
  (not light)
2 teaspoons baking powder
1 teaspoon sugar
½ teaspoon baking soda
¼–½ teaspoon salt, to taste
1 cup nonfat buttermilk
Cooking spray
2 tablespoons plus 2 teaspoons
  strawberry all-fruit spread

1. Preheat oven to 450°F.
2. In a food processor, combine flour, margarine, baking powder, sugar, baking soda, and salt. Process to a coarse meal texture. Place flour mixture in a mixing bowl, make a well in center, and add buttermilk. Stir lightly until *just* blended; *do not* overmix.
3. Coat a nonstick baking sheet with cooking spray. Spoon mixture onto baking sheet in 12 mounds. Bake for 12 minutes and serve immediately. Allow two biscuits and 2 teaspoons strawberry spread for serving. Remaining biscuits may be stored for up to two days in an airtight container at room temperature.

SCRAMBLED EGGS *(52 calories, 0.2 g fat per serving)*

2 8-ounce cartons egg substitute
½ teaspoon Worcestershire sauce
⅛ teaspoon salt
⅛ teaspoon black pepper or to
  taste
Dash cayenne pepper
Cooking spray

Whisk together all ingredients except cooking spray. Liberally coat a large nonstick skillet with spray and place over medium-high heat for 1 minute. Add egg mixture. When edges begin to get firm, push eggs to center with a spatula, allowing uncooked portion to cook. Gently turn eggs to desired doneness. Serve immediately.

CANADIAN BACON *(70 calories, 2 g fat per serving)*

8 1-ounce slices Oscar Mayer 93
  percent fat-free Canadian
  bacon

1. Preheat oven to warm.
2. Set bacon on an ovenproof platter, place in oven, heat until warm (3–5 minutes). Remove from oven and serve.

(Continued on the next page)

GRAPEFRUIT *(43 calories, 0 g fat per serving)*

2 large maraschino cherries, halved
2 medium-sized grapefruit (any variety)

Cut grapefruits in half. Top each with a cherry half and serve.

CAMP-STYLE POTATO PATTIES WITH BACON, TOAST, AND FRESH PEACH SLICES

Serves 4

Total calories per serving: 350
Total fat per serving: 5.7 g (15%)

CAMP-STYLE POTATO PATTIES WITH BACON (259 calories, 5.7 g fat per serving)

8 slices Oscar Mayer 93 percent fat-free bacon
1 quart water
1 pound unpeeled white potatoes, cut into 1-inch pieces
¼ cup finely chopped yellow onion
1 large egg white
¼ cup evaporated skim milk
1 tablespoon light margarine
½ teaspoon salt
⅛ teaspoon black pepper
3 tablespoons plus 1½ teaspoons all-purpose flour
Butter-flavored cooking spray
2 teaspoons vegetable oil

1. Preheat broiler.
2. Place bacon on a broiler rack and broil until crisp (about 3 minutes). Transfer to a paper towel–lined ovenproof platter. Reset oven to warm. Place bacon in oven.
3. In a medium-sized saucepan, bring water to a boil and add potatoes. Return to a boil, reduce heat, and simmer for 20 minutes or until tender. Drain well. Place in a mixing bowl and beat until fairly smooth using an electric mixer. Add onion, egg white, evaporated milk, margarine, salt, and pepper. Beat until well blended. Beat in flour.
4. Coat a large nonstick skillet with cooking spray, add 1 teaspoon vegetable oil, spread around bottom of pan to coat evenly, and place over medium-high heat for 1½ minutes. Using half of the potato mixture, spoon four mounds into skillet and flatten using back of a fork to form 4-inch patties. Cook for 6 minutes, turn, and cook for 5–6 minutes longer. Transfer to a plate and place in warm oven. Repeat with remaining oil and potato mixture. Serve immediately.

TOAST (54 calories, 0 g fat per serving)

4 slices light bread
4 teaspoons all-fruit spread (any flavor)

Toast bread. Top each slice with 1 teaspoon spread and serve.

FRESH PEACH SLICES (37 calories, 0 g fat per serving)

4 medium-sized peaches

Rinse peaches. Peel, if desired, and cut each peach into eights, discarding pits. Serve eight slices on each of four small plates.

BLUEBERRY SHORTCAKE COBBLER, CANADIAN BACON, AND COLD MILK

Serves 4

Total calories per serving: 350
Total fat per serving: 4.9 g (13%)

BLUEBERRY SHORTCAKE COBBLER *(229 calories, 3 g fat per serving)*

½ cup plus 1 tablespoon all-purpose flour
2 teaspoons margarine (not light)
2½ tablespoons sugar
½ teaspoon baking powder
⅛ teaspoon baking soda
⅓ cup nonfat buttermilk
Cooking spray
1 1-pound bag frozen unsweetened blueberries, thawed
2 tablespoons frozen grape juice concentrate
1 tablespoon cornstarch
½ teaspoon vanilla extract

1. Preheat oven to 450°F.
2. In a food processor, combine flour, margarine, 1 tablespoon sugar, baking powder, and baking soda. Process to a coarse meal texture. Transfer to a mixing bowl, add buttermilk, and mix gently until *just* blended.
3. Coat an 8-inch square nonstick baking pan with cooking spray. Add blueberries, juice concentrate, cornstarch, remaining 1½ tablespoons sugar, and vanilla to pan. Stir until cornstarch dissolves. Spoon batter on top of berries in four mounds and bake for 20–25 minutes or until lightly browned. Remove and let stand for 5 minutes before spooning into bowls to serve.

CANADIAN BACON *(53 calories, 1.5 g fat per serving)*

6 1-ounce slices Oscar Mayer 93 percent fat-free Canadian bacon

1. Preheat oven to warm.
2. Set bacon on an ovenproof plate, place in oven, and heat until warm (3–5 minutes). Remove from oven and serve.

COLD MILK *(68 calories, 0.4 g fat per serving)*

3 cups skim milk, chilled

Serve ¾ cup milk in each of four glasses.

BUTTERMILK PANCAKES WITH BLUEBERRY SAUCE, CANADIAN BACON, AND SLICED FRESH ORANGES

Serves 4

Total calories per serving: 348
Total fat per serving: 7 g (18%)

BUTTERMILK PANCAKES *(201 calories, 4.5 g fat per serving)*

1 cup plus 2 tablespoons all-purpose flour
2 tablespoons sugar
1 teaspoon baking powder
¼ teaspoon baking soda
¼ teaspoon salt
1 cup plus 7 tablespoons nonfat buttermilk
1 tablespoon vegetable oil
1 large egg
1 large egg white
2 teaspoons vanilla extract
Cooking spray

1. Preheat oven to warm.
2. In a mixing bowl, combine flour, sugar, baking powder, baking soda, and salt. Mix thoroughly and set aside.
3. In a separate bowl, combine buttermilk, oil, egg, egg white, and vanilla; whisk to blend *thoroughly*. Make a well in center of dry ingredients, add buttermilk mixture, and stir gently, using a rubber spatula, until *just* blended; batter will be lumpy.
4. Coat a large nonstick skillet with cooking spray and place over medium-high heat for 1½ minutes. Using 2½ tablespoons batter for each pancake, spoon batter onto skillet and cook for 1½ minutes or until bubbles begin to appear. Turn and cook for about 1 minute. Transfer to a serving platter and place in warm oven. Repeat until all batter is used. Place three pancakes on each plate and top with one-fourth of sauce.

BLUEBERRY SAUCE *(46 calories, 0.5 g fat per serving)*

1 cup frozen unsweetened blueberries
¼ cup unsweetened grape juice
1 tablespoon sugar
1½ teaspoons cornstarch
½ teaspoon vanilla extract

In a small saucepan, combine frozen blueberries, grape juice, sugar, and cornstarch. Stir until cornstarch dissolves. Bring to a boil, stirring frequently, and continue boiling for 1 minute. Stir well, remove from heat and stir in vanilla. Before serving, sauce may be reheated if desired.

(Continued on the next page)

CANADIAN BACON *(70 calories, 2 g fat per serving)*

8 1-ounce slices Oscar Mayer 93 percent fat-free Canadian bacon

1. Preheat oven to warm.
2. Set bacon on an ovenproof platter and place in oven until warm (3–5 minutes). Remove from oven and serve.

SLICED FRESH ORANGES *(31 calories, 0 g fat per serving)*

2 medium-sized oranges, peeled   Cut each orange into 8 slices and serve.

CINNAMON SHORTCAKES WITH FRESH PEACHES, VANILLA CREAM, AND HAM SLICES

Serves 4

Total calories per serving: 340
Total fat per serving: 6.9 g (18%)

CINNAMON SHORTCAKES WITH FRESH PEACHES *(213 calories, 4.7 g fat per serving)*

1 cup plus 2 tablespoons Bisquick
  Reduced Fat baking mix
2 tablespoons sugar
½ teaspoon ground cinnamon
⅛ teaspoon ground nutmeg
6 tablespoons skim milk
2 tablespoons light margarine,
  melted
Cooking spray
2 cups sliced fresh peaches

1. Preheat oven to 450°F.
2. In a mixing bowl, combine baking mix, sugar, cinnamon, and nutmeg; blend thoroughly. Add milk and melted margarine and stir until *just* blended. Coat a nonstick baking sheet with cooking spray and spoon batter onto sheet in four mounds. Bake for 10–12 minutes or until lightly browned.
3. Place shortcakes in four bowls. Spoon ½ cup sliced peaches over each shortcake and top with one-fourth of the Vanilla Cream.

VANILLA CREAM *(53 calories, 0.2 g fat per serving)*

1 cup skim milk
1 tablespoon cornstarch
2 tablespoons sugar
1 tablespoon vanilla extract

In a medium-sized saucepan, whisk together milk and cornstarch until cornstarch dissolves. Stir in sugar until well blended. Place over medium-high heat and cook until thickened, stirring with a spatula. Remove from heat and add vanilla. Chill thoroughly.

Variation: This may be made the night before.

HAM SLICES *(74 calories, 2 g fat per serving)*

8 1-ounce slices extra-lean ham

1. Preheat oven to warm.
2. Place ham on an ovenproof platter and set in oven. Heat for 3–4 minutes. Remove from oven and serve.

PANFRIED STEAK AND HASH BROWN POTATOES

Serves 4

Total calories per serving: 341
Total fat per serving: 10 g (26%)

PANFRIED STEAK *(153 calories, 5.1 g fat per serving)*

Cooking spray
1 pound top round, trimmed of
    all fat and cut into 4 pieces
¼ teaspoon garlic powder
Black pepper to taste
1 teaspoon Worcestershire sauce

Coat a large skillet with cooking spray and place over high heat for 1 minute. Add two pieces of steak and sprinkle with ⅛ teaspoon garlic powder and black pepper. Cook for 2 minutes, turn steaks, reduce heat to medium, and cook for 2–3 minutes longer, or until steaks are cooked as desired. Spoon ¼ teaspoon Worcestershire sauce over each steak and sprinkle with more black pepper. Place in a warm oven and repeat with remaining steak.

HASH BROWN POTATOES *(188 calories, 4.9 g fat per serving)*

14 ounces unpeeled red potatoes,
    shredded (about 3 cups)
⅔ cup chopped yellow onion
2 large egg whites
¼ cup all-purpose flour
¼ teaspoon salt
⅛ teaspoon cayenne pepper
⅛ teaspoon black pepper
Butter-flavored cooking spray
1 tablespoon plus 1 teaspoon
    margarine (not light)
1 teaspoon vegetable oil

1. Preheat oven to warm.
2. Dry potatoes and onions with paper towels, pressing out any excess moisture. Toss with egg whites, flour, salt, cayenne, and black pepper; mix well.
3. Coat a large nonstick skillet with cooking spray. Add 2 teaspoons of the margarine and ½ teaspoon of the oil to skillet and place over medium-high heat. When margarine begins to bubble, spoon half of the potato mixture in four mounds onto skillet. Flatten each to form a 4-inch patty. Cook for 4 minutes, turn, and cook for 5 minutes longer. Place on a platter in warm oven and repeat with remaining margarine, oil, and potato mixture.

CHEESE GRITS, BROILED TOMATOES, WARM BAGELS, AND FRESH MELON

Serves 4

Total calories per serving: 349
Total fat per serving: 7.1 g (18%)

CHEESE GRITS *(153 calories, 4 g fat per serving)*

1 quart water
⅔ cup (¼ pound) uncooked quick grits
3 ounces Velveeta Light cheese, cut into ½-inch pieces
1 teaspoon Worcestershire sauce
½ teaspoon salt
⅛ teaspoon cayenne pepper
⅛ teaspoon garlic powder (if desired)

In a medium-sized saucepan, bring water to a boil, stir in grits, reduce heat, and simmer, uncovered, for 5 minutes, stirring occasionally. Remove from heat and stir in cheese, Worcestershire, salt, cayenne, and garlic powder if desired. Cover and let stand for 3 minutes. Stir and serve.

BROILED TOMATOES *(43 calories, 0.3 g fat per serving)*

4 medium-sized tomatoes, halved crosswise
1 tablespoon plus 1 teaspoon fresh lemon juice
1 slice light bread, toasted and grated
2 tablespoons finely chopped fresh parsley
⅛ teaspoon salt
Freshly ground black pepper to taste
Olive oil–flavored or butter-flavored cooking spray

1. Preheat the broiler.
2. Place tomato halves on broiler pan cut side up. Spoon ½ teaspoon lemon juice over each half. In a small bowl, combine bread crumbs, parsley, salt, and pepper. Toss well and sprinkle evenly over tomato halves. Spray lightly with cooking spray. Place in broiler no less than 5 inches from heat source. Broil for 3 minutes. Turn heat off, letting tomatoes remain in oven for 4 minutes longer.

(Continued on the next page)

WARM BAGELS *(95 calories, 2.5 g fat per serving)*

2 bagels (plain, egg, or rye)
4 teaspoons light margarine

Split bagels and toast halves. Spread 1 teaspoon margarine over each half and serve.

FRESH MELON *(58 calories, 0.3 g fat per serving)*

2 cups cubed cantaloupe
2 cups cubed honeydew

Combine fruits. Serve one-quarter of mixture in each of four small bowls.

DOWN-HOME TOMATO GRAVY AND GRITS, CANADIAN BACON, TOAST, AND FRESH MELON SLICES

Serves 4

Total calories per serving: 339
Total fat per serving: 6.8 g (18%)

DOWN-HOME TOMATO GRAVY AND GRITS (195 calories, 4.7 g fat per serving)

1 slice lower-sodium bacon
1¼ cups skim milk
2 tablespoons all-purpose flour
1 16-ounce can tomatoes,
    undrained, chopped
¼ teaspoon salt
⅛ teaspoon sugar
Black pepper to taste
3 cups cooked grits, no salt or
    margarine used in cooking

1. Place bacon in a skillet, preferably cast iron, over medium heat, cook until crisp, remove bacon, and set aside.
2. In a separate bowl, whisk together milk and flour until well blended. Slowly whisk mixture into drippings in skillet. Blend thoroughly. Stir in tomatoes, their liquid, salt, sugar, and black pepper. Cook, stirring occasionally with a spatula, for 25 minutes. Spoon ¾ cup grits onto each plate and top with one-fourth of the tomato gravy.

CANADIAN BACON (70 calories, 2 g fat per serving)

8 1-ounce slices Oscar Mayer 93
    **percent fat-free Canadian
    bacon**

1. Preheat oven to warm.
2. Set bacon on an ovenproof platter, place in oven, and heat until warm (3–5 minutes). Remove from oven and serve.

TOAST (54 calories, 0 g fat per serving)

4 slices light bread
4 teaspoons all-fruit spread (any
    flavor)

Toast bread. Top each slice with 1 teaspoon spread and serve.

FRESH MELON SLICES (20 calories, 0.1 g fat per serving)

½ medium-sized cantaloupe

Cut cantaloupe into four even wedges and serve.

FRESH TOMATO AND PROVOLONE PIZZA QUICHE

Serves 4

Total calories per serving: 348
Total fat per serving: 9.5 g (25%)

Olive-oil–flavored cooking spray
1 10-ounce can refrigerated pizza crust dough
1 teaspoon extra-virgin olive oil
4 cloves garlic, minced
1 cup thinly sliced onion
½ cup (2 ounces) grated smoked provolone cheese
½ cup (2 ounces) grated part-skim mozzarella cheese
1 tablespoon plus 1 teaspoon freshly grated Parmesan cheese
3 plum tomatoes, cut into ¼-inch slices
¾ teaspoon dried basil leaves
½ cup egg substitute
½ cup nonfat cottage cheese
½ cup evaporated skim milk
2 tablespoons chopped fresh parsley
¼ teaspoon black pepper

1. Preheat oven to 350°F.

2. Coat a 9″ × 13″ baking pan with cooking spray. Lightly press dough into bottom and ½ inch up sides of baking pan and set aside. Coat a nonstick skillet with cooking spray, add olive oil, and heat over medium heat for 1 minute. Add garlic and cook for 15 seconds. Add onion and cook, stirring occasionally, for about 8 minutes or until beginning to brown. Arrange evenly on dough. Sprinkle provolone, mozzarella, and Parmesan cheeses over onion. Evenly space tomato slices over cheeses and sprinkle with basil.

3. In a food processor, combine egg substitute, cottage cheese, evaporated milk, parsley, and pepper. Process until smooth and carefully pour over all.

4. Bake for 30 minutes. Transfer to a wire rack and let stand for 10 minutes before serving.

CHERRY CRUMBLE AND CINNAMON-VANILLA YOGURT

Serves 4

Total calories per serving: 349
Total fat per serving: 5.2 g (13%)

CHERRY CRUMBLE *(249 calories, 5.2 g fat per serving)*

¾ cup quick-cooking oats
6 tablespoons all-purpose flour
¼ cup sugar
1 teaspoon ground cinnamon
½ teaspoon baking powder
¼ teaspoon baking soda
⅛ teaspoon salt
¼ cup cold light margarine
1 16-ounce can pitted sour
    cherries, undrained
1 tablespoon plus 1 teaspoon
    cornstarch
2 teaspoons vanilla extract
Cooking spray

1. Preheat oven to 350°F.
2. In a food processor, combine oats, flour, 3 tablespoons of the sugar, ½ teaspoon of the cinnamon, the baking powder, baking soda, salt, and margarine. Process, pulsing, until mixture has a coarse meal texture.
3. In a small saucepan, combine cherries with liquid, cornstarch, and remaining 1 tablespoon sugar. Stir until cornstarch dissolves. Bring to a boil and continue boiling for 1 minute, stirring occasionally. Remove from heat and stir in vanilla.
4. Coat an 8-inch square pan with cooking spray. Spoon cherry mixture into pan, top with crumbled oat mixture, and sprinkle with remaining ½ teaspoon cinnamon. Bake for 30 minutes. Serve warm or at room temperature.

CINNAMON-VANILLA YOGURT *(100 calories, 0 g fat per serving)*

4 cups vanilla nonfat yogurt
1½ teaspoons cinnamon

Combine yogurt and cinnamon. Serve 1 cup of mixture in each of four small bowls.

PUFFED BLINTZES WITH RICH CHEESECAKE SAUCE AND RASPBERRIES AND MIXED FRUIT SMOOTHIES

Serves 4

Total calories per serving: 330
Total fat per serving: 2.9 g (8%)

PUFFED BLINTZES WITH RICH CHEESECAKE SAUCE AND RASPBERRIES
(168 calories, 1.7 g fat per serving)

Rich Cheesecake Sauce and Raspberries
½ cup (4 ounces) fat-free cream cheese
2 tablespoons powdered sugar
1 tablespoon skim milk
1 teaspoon vanilla extract
½ cup frozen raspberries in light syrup, thawed

Puffed Blintzes
Cooking spray
⅔ cup low-fat (1½ percent) buttermilk
½ cup all-purpose flour
1 tablespoon sugar
1 teaspoon grated orange zest
1 large egg
1 large egg white

1. In a food processor, combine cream cheese, powdered sugar, milk, and vanilla. Process until smooth. Set sauce and raspberries aside until blintzes are ready to serve.
2. Preheat oven to 425°F. Coat a 9-inch pie pan with cooking spray.
3. In a food processor, combine buttermilk, flour, sugar, zest, egg, and egg white. Process until smooth and quickly pour into pie pan. Bake for 18 minutes or until golden and puffy. Transfer pan to a wire rack.
4. When puff settles, cut into four wedges and place on four plates. Spoon equal amounts of sauce onto center of each wedge and top with raspberries and syrup.

MIXED FRUIT SMOOTHIES *(162 calories, 1.2 g fat per serving)*

3 cups skim milk
2 medium-sized bananas
2 cups strawberries, rinsed and hulled
1 tablespoon plus 1 teaspoon honey

In a blender, blend together all ingredients. Serve in tall glasses.

PECAN CARAMEL COFFEE CAKE, FRESH MELON, AND COLD MILK

Serves 4

Total calories per serving: 326
Total fat per serving: 7.6 g (21%)

PECAN CARAMEL COFFEE CAKE *(200 calories, 6.8 g fat per serving)*

1½ cups all-purpose flour
⅓ cup quick-cooking oats
⅓ cup granulated sugar
1 tablespoon baking powder
½ teaspoon baking soda
1 teaspoon ground cinnamon
¼ teaspoon salt
¼ cup natural applesauce
1 tablespoon plus 1½ teaspoons
    vegetable oil
¾ cup skim milk
1 large egg
½ teaspoon vanilla butter nut
    flavoring
Cooking spray
3 tablespoons dark brown sugar
3 tablespoons light margarine
¼ cup (1 ounce) pecan pieces,
    toasted in broiler

1. Preheat oven to 375°F.
2. In a food processor, combine 1¼ cups flour, oats, granulated sugar, baking powder, baking soda, ½ teaspoon cinnamon, and salt. Process until fine. Transfer to a mixing bowl and set aside. Place applesauce, oil, milk, egg, and flavoring in processor and blend well.
3. Make a well in center of dry ingredients and add applesauce mixture. Stir *just* until blended; do *not* overmix. Pour batter into a 9-inch square baking pan coated with cooking spray. Bake for 25 minutes or until a toothpick inserted in center comes out clean. Place on a wire rack and let stand for 5 minutes.
4. Meanwhile, in processor, combine brown sugar, margarine, remaining ¼ cup flour, and remaining ½ teaspoon cinnamon. Process until it forms a paste, then spread paste over cake. Sprinkle with pecans.
5. Cut cake into nine 3-inch-square servings. Place one square on each of four plates and serve warm or at room temperature. Remaining cake may be stored in an airtight container for up to four days at room temperature.

FRESH MELON *(58 calories, 0.3 g fat per serving)*

2 cups cubed cantaloupe
2 cups cubed honeydew

Combine fruits. Serve one-quarter of mixture in each of four small bowls.

COLD MILK *(68 calories, 0.4 g fat per serving)*

3 cups skim milk, chilled

Serve ¾ cup milk in each of four glasses.

FRESH BANANA–OAT BREAD AND VANILLA YOGURT WITH SLICED FRESH PEACHES

Serves 4

Total calories per serving: 340
Total fat per serving: 6.6 g (17%)

FRESH BANANA–OAT BREAD (254 calories, 6.6 g fat per serving)

1 cup all-purpose flour
⅔ cup quick-cooking oats
⅓ cup sugar
1 tablespoon baking powder
½ teaspoon baking soda
1 teaspoon ground cinnamon
½ teaspoon ground nutmeg
⅛ teaspoon salt
1 cup nonfat buttermilk
1 large egg
2 tablespoons vegetable oil
2 teaspoons vanilla extract
2 *very ripe* medium-sized
    bananas, mashed (about 1 cup)
Cooking spray

1. Preheat oven to 350°F.
2. In a mixing bowl, combine flour, oats, sugar, baking powder, baking soda, cinnamon, nutmeg, and salt. Blend thoroughly and set aside.
3. In a separate bowl, whisk together buttermilk, egg, oil, and vanilla. Add bananas and mix thoroughly. Make a well in center of dry ingredients. Add liquid ingredients and stir gently until *just* blended; do *not* overmix.
4. Coat a nonstick 9″ × 5″ loaf pan with cooking spray. Pour batter into pan and bake for 50 minutes. Immediately remove from pan and place on a wire rack to cool for 10 minutes before cutting into 12 slices. Serve warm or at room temperature. Allow two slices per serving. Remaining bread may be stored in an airtight container for up to four days at room temperature.

Variation: For quick muffins: Pour batter into 12 muffin cups and bake for 20 minutes. Let stand for 2–3 minutes before removing from tin. Allow two muffins per serving.

VANILLA YOGURT WITH SLICED FRESH PEACHES (86 calories, 0 g fat per serving)

2 cups sliced peaches
2 cups vanilla nonfat yogurt
Ground cinnamon for garnish

Place ½ cup peach slices on each of 4 small plates. Top each with ½ cup yogurt. Sprinkle lightly with cinnamon and serve.

BLUEBERRY-OATMEAL MUFFINS
AND SLICED BANANAS WITH VANILLA YOGURT

Serves 4

Total calories per serving: 336
Total fat per serving: 5.8 g (16%)

BLUEBERRY-OATMEAL MUFFINS *(253 calories, 5.5 g fat per serving)*

1¼ cups all-purpose flour
⅔ cup quick-cooking oats
½ cup sugar
1 tablespoon baking powder
½ teaspoon baking soda
¼ teaspoon salt
1 cup nonfat buttermilk
2 tablespoons vegetable oil
1 tablespoon vanilla extract
2 large egg whites
1 cup blueberries, thawed if
   frozen
Cooking spray

1. Preheat oven to 400°F.
2. In a medium-sized mixing bowl, combine flour, oats, sugar, baking powder, baking soda, and salt. Blend thoroughly and set aside.
3. In a separate bowl, combine buttermilk, oil, vanilla, and egg whites. Blend thoroughly. Make a well in center of dry ingredients and add wet ingredients and blueberries. Gently mix until *just* blended.
4. Coat a nonstick 12-cup muffin tin with cooking spray and gently spoon equal amounts of batter into the cups. Bake for 18 minutes. Let stand for 2–3 minutes before removing from tin. Allow two muffins per serving. Remaining muffins may be stored for up to four days in an airtight container at room temperature.

SLICED BANANAS WITH VANILLA YOGURT *(83 calories, 0.3 g fat per serving)*

2 medium-sized bananas, sliced
1⅓ cups vanilla nonfat yogurt
Ground nutmeg for garnish

Place one-fourth of the banana slices in each of four small bowls. Top each with ⅓ cup yogurt. Sprinkle lightly with nutmeg and serve.

PECAN-PUMPKIN BRAN MUFFINS AND FRUIT WITH SPICED ORANGE CREAM

Serves 4

Total calories per serving: 343
Total fat per serving: 8.8 g (23%)

PECAN-PUMPKIN BRAN MUFFINS *(228 calories, 8.5 g fat per serving)*

1 cup All-Bran with Extra Fiber cereal
1¼ cups nonfat buttermilk
1 cup all-purpose flour
7 tablespoons sugar
1 tablespoon baking powder
½ teaspoon baking soda
¼ teaspoon salt
1 tablespoon apple pie spice
2 tablespoons vegetable oil
1 large egg, well beaten
1 tablespoon vanilla extract
1 cup canned pumpkin
Cooking spray
⅓ cup (1½ ounces) pecan pieces
½ teaspoon ground cinnamon

1. Preheat oven to 400°F.
2. In a mixing bowl, combine bran and buttermilk; stir to moisten and let stand for 5 minutes.
3. In a separate bowl, combine flour, 5 tablespoons sugar, baking powder, baking soda, salt, and apple pie spice. Blend thoroughly. To bran mixture, add oil, egg, vanilla, and pumpkin. Mix well. Make a well in center of dry ingredients and pour pumpkin mixture into it; stir gently until *just* blended.
4. Coat a nonstick muffin tin or tins with at least 15 cups with cooking spray and spoon batter into 15 cups. Sprinkle pecans evenly over muffins. In a small container, combine remaining 2 tablespoons sugar with cinnamon. Mix well and sprinkle over pecans. Bake for 20 minutes. Remove immediately and place on wire racks. Let stand for 5 minutes to finish cooking on racks. Serve warm or at room temperature. Allow two muffins per serving. Remaining muffins may be stored for up to four days in an airtight container at room temperature.

FRUIT WITH SPICED ORANGE CREAM *(115 calories, 0.3 g fat per serving)*

½ cup nonfat sour cream
1 tablespoon dark brown sugar
¼ teaspoon ground ginger
Dash ground nutmeg
½ teaspoon grated orange zest
½ cup juice-packed canned pineapple chunks, drained
1 cup seedless red or green grapes, halved
1 cup sliced bananas

1. In a small bowl, combine sour cream, brown sugar, ginger, nutmeg, and orange zest. Blend well and chill.
2. At serving time, combine fruits and divide among individual plates. Top each with 2 tablespoons sauce and serve immediately.

BOUNTIFUL FRUITS AND CEREAL, TOAST, AND CHILLED TOMATO JUICE

Serves 4

Total calories per serving: 349
Total fat per serving: 3.3 g (9%)

BOUNTIFUL FRUITS AND CEREAL *(249 calories, 1.3 g fat per serving)*

4 cups Total corn or wheat flakes
1 cup sliced bananas
1 cup sliced peaches
1 cup sliced strawberries
1 cup blueberries
3 cups skim milk
4 teaspoons sugar

Place 1 cup cereal in each of four cereal bowls. Top each with ¼ cup each bananas, peaches, strawberries, and blueberries. Pour ¾ cup milk over each serving and top with 1 teaspoon sugar. Serve immediately.

TOAST *(65 calories, 2 g fat per serving)*

4 slices light bread
4 teaspoons light margarine

Toast bread. Spread 1 teaspoon margarine on each slice and serve.

CHILLED TOMATO JUICE *(35 calories, 0 g fat per serving)*

3 cups tomato juice, chilled

Serve ¾ cup juice in each of four glasses.

CITRUS-SWEETENED FRUIT WITH APRICOT-TOPPED ENGLISH MUFFINS

Serves 4

Total calories per serving: 348
Total fat per serving: 2.4 g (6%)

CITRUS-SWEETENED FRUIT *(134 calories, 1.3 g fat per serving)*

4 medium-sized nectarines,
   pitted and sliced thin
35 dark sweet cherries (about 1¾
   cups), halved and pitted, *or* 2¾
   cups seedless red grapes,
   halved
¼ cup frozen pineapple-orange
   juice concentrate
⅛ teaspoon ground ginger
⅛ teaspoon ground nutmeg

Place sliced nectarines and cherries in a decorative bowl. Combine juice concentrate with ginger and nutmeg and blend thoroughly. Add to fruit, toss well, and chill for 30 minutes.

APRICOT-TOPPED ENGLISH MUFFINS *(214 calories, 1.1 g fat per serving)*

¼ cup apricot all-fruit spread
½ cup fat-free cream cheese
4 English muffins, halved and
   toasted

In a small saucepan over low heat, heat apricot spread until melted. Spread 1 tablespoon cream cheese on each muffin half and spoon 1½ teaspoons of the apricot spread on top of cream cheese. Serve immediately.

INDIVIDUAL FRUIT PLATTERS WITH HOT POPOVERS

Serves 4   **Total calories per serving: 350**
           Total fat per serving: 4 g (10%)

INDIVIDUAL FRUIT PLATTERS (154 calories, 0.6 g fat per serving)

⅓ cup raspberry or apricot all-
   fruit spread
1 cup sliced fresh peaches
1 cup cubed honeydew
1 cup seedless red grapes
1 cup cubed cantaloupe
1 cup quartered strawberries
1 cup cubed watermelon, seeded
¾ cup blueberries

In a small saucepan over medium-low heat, melt fruit spread. Do *not* bring to a boil. On individual plates, spoon 1 tablespoon plus 1 teaspoon of the spread and spread evenly to coat a 6-inch area using back of a spoon. Decoratively arrange ¼ cup each peaches, honeydew, grapes, cantaloupe, and strawberries around outer edges of plates. Place ¼ cup watermelon and 3 tablespoons blueberries in center.

POPOVERS (196 calories, 3.4 g fat per serving)

4 large egg whites
1 cup skim milk
1⅓ cups all-purpose flour
¼ teaspoon salt
2 tablespoons plus 2 teaspoons
   light margarine

1. Preheat oven to 450°F.
2. In a mixing bowl, whisk together egg whites and milk until well blended. Gradually add flour and salt and stir lightly until *just* blended. Do not overmix. Place a nonstick muffin tin with at least 8 cups in oven for 3 minutes. Remove, immediately coat with cooking spray, and spoon batter evenly into eight of the cups. Bake for 15 minutes, reduce heat to 350°F, and bake for 25 minutes longer. Serve immediately with margarine.

LUNCHES

❧

Lunch Counter BLT–Tuna Salad Club and Fresh Peach Slices

Curried Tuna and Pecans in Pita Halves with Ambrosia Fruits

Shrimp and Pasta Salad with Fresh Ripe Tomatoes

Shrimp and Cheese Chowder

Stacked Turkey Sandwiches, Green Pea Salad, and Cranberry Spritzer

Sugar-Glazed Chicken and Orange-Curry Salad with Peanuts

Cantaloupe Halves Stuffed with Curried Chicken Salad

Chicken with Lime Creole Sauce in Tortillas

Chicken and Pepperoncini Salad with Feta and Fresh Croutons

Louisiana Blackened Chicken Salad with Toasted Cajun Bread

Quick Italian Beef Pizza Bread and Simple Tossed Salad with Parmesan

Roast Beef Salad with Blue Cheese in Pitas and Sliced Fresh Apples

Hamburgers on Toasted Buns with Pickle Spears

Wild Rice–Sausage Chowder and Fresh Tomato Slices

*Hearty Sausage and Pasta Stew and Mixed Greens with
Creamy Lemon Garlic Dressing*

Ham, Tomato, and Sprout Sandwiches, Potato Salad, and Orange Fresher

Fireside White Bean and Sausage Soup with Simple Spiced Italian Salad

Rolled Ham with Cream Cheese and Sweet Red Poppy Fruit–Lettuce Platter

Stuffed Potatoes with Vegetables, Cheese, and Bacon, Sour Cream–Scallion Salad, and Sliced Fresh Apples

Ham Slices with Sweet Curry, Fruit, and Rice Salad and Melba Rounds with Cream Cheese

Fresh Garden Ravioli and Mozzarella Soup with Asparagus Spear Salad

Bean and Cheese Tostadas, Simple Peppered Salad, and Limeade

Hot Open-Faced Cheese Sandwiches and Raspberry-Wine Vinaigrette Salad

Jalapeño-Cheese Corn Bread Squares with Salsa and Sliced Cucumbers with Sour Cream Dressing

Egg Salad Sandwiches, Sliced Fresh Apples, and Chilled Gazpacho with Fresh Cilantro

Winter Vegetable Soup, Garlic Italian Bread, and Cinnamon-Dusted Apple Slices

Mediterranean Couscous Salad with Fresh Limes, Cucumbers, and Tomatoes

Three-Rice Salad with Almonds and Peas

Peppered Lime Soup, Mozzarella Tortilla Wedges, and Black-Eyed Pea Salad

Spiced Jamaican Chili with Rice

LUNCH COUNTER BLT–TUNA SALAD CLUB
AND FRESH PEACH SLICES

Serves 4

Total calories per serving: 343
Total fat per serving: 10.6 g (28%)

LUNCH COUNTER BLT–TUNA SALAD CLUB *(306 calories, 10.6 g fat per serving)*

2 6-ounce cans water-packed
   tuna
5 tablespoons fat-free
   mayonnaise-style salad dressing
4 hard-cooked eggs
½ cup thinly sliced celery
1 tablespoon plus 1 teaspoon
   sweet pickle relish
1 teaspoon sugar
¼ teaspoon black pepper
8 slices light bread, toasted
4 lettuce leaves
4 slices tomato
4 slices lower-sodium bacon,
   broiled and halved

Place tuna in a colander, rinse with water, and drain well, shaking out any excess water. Place in a bowl, mix with 2 tablespoons plus 1 teaspoon salad dressing, and set aside. Chop two eggs and add to tuna. Discard yolks of remaining two eggs. Chop two egg whites and add to tuna along with celery, relish, sugar, and pepper. Blend well. At serving time, spread 1 teaspoon of remaining mayonnaise on each slice of toast. Top four slices with a lettuce leaf, a slice of tomato, one-fourth of the tuna mixture, and two slices of bacon. Place four remaining slices of toast on top. Cut each sandwich into fourths, secure with toothpicks, and serve immediately.

FRESH PEACH SLICES *(37 calories, 0 g fat per serving)*

4 medium-sized peaches

Peel peaches, if desired. Cut each into eight wedges, discarding pits. Serve one-fourth slices on each of four small plates.

CURRIED TUNA AND PECANS IN PITA HALVES WITH AMBROSIA FRUITS

Serves 4

Total calories per serving: 349
Total fat per serving: 9.9 g (26%)

CURRIED TUNA AND PECANS IN PITA HALVES *(247 calories, 8.1 g fat per serving)*

2 6-ounce cans water-packed
   tuna
½ cup fat-free mayonnaise-style
   salad dressing
¼ cup thinly sliced celery
2 tablespoons sweet pickle relish
2 teaspoons curry powder
½ teaspoon sugar
⅜ teaspoon black pepper
¼ cup pecan pieces, toasted in
   broiler
2 loaves pita, halved to make
   pockets
4 Boston lettuce leaves

Place tuna in a colander, rinse with water, and drain well, shaking out any excess water. Place in a bowl and add salad dressing, celery, relish, curry powder, sugar, and pepper; blend well. Stir in pecans. At serving time, line pita halves with lettuce leaves and fill each half with one-fourth of the tuna mixture.

AMBROSIA FRUITS *(102 calories, 1.8 g fat per serving)*

4 medium-sized oranges,
   sectioned and halved
1 cup strawberries, quartered
½ cup seedless green grapes
½ medium-sized pink grapefruit,
   sectioned and halved
3 tablespoons sweetened flaked
   coconut
¼ teaspoon coconut extract

Combine all ingredients and toss gently but thoroughly.

SHRIMP AND PASTA SALAD WITH FRESH RIPE TOMATOES

Serves 4

Total calories per serving: 349
Total fat per serving: 3.4 g (9%)

2½ cups peeled cooked shrimp, chilled (about 18 ounces)
3 cups cooled cooked penne, no butter, margarine, or oil used in cooking
1 14-ounce can artichoke hearts, well drained and quartered
¼ cup finely chopped yellow onion
¼ cup chopped fresh parsley
¾ cup fat-free mayonnaise-style salad dressing
¼ cup fresh lemon juice
1 clove garlic, minced
½ teaspoon dried oregano leaves
½ teaspoon dried basil leaves
½ teaspoon salt
¼ teaspoon black pepper
¼ teaspoon paprika
2 tablespoons plus 2 teaspoons freshly grated Parmesan cheese
4 lettuce leaves
Freshly ground black pepper to taste
4 medium-sized tomatoes, each cut into 8 wedges

1. In a medium-sized mixing bowl, combine shrimp, pasta, artichoke hearts, onions, and parsley. Set aside.

2. In a separate bowl, combine salad dressing, 3 tablespoons lemon juice, garlic, oregano, basil, ¼ teaspoon salt, pepper, and paprika. Blend thoroughly and spoon over shrimp mixture. Toss gently but thoroughly to coat. Chill for 1 hour.

3. At serving time, add remaining tablespoon of lemon juice and remaining ¼ teaspoon salt. Add Parmesan and toss again. Spoon one-fourth of shrimp onto a bed of lettuce, sprinkle lightly with freshly ground pepper, and arrange eight tomato wedges around each serving. Serve immediately.

SHRIMP AND CHEESE CHOWDER

Serves 4

Total calories per serving: 347
Total fat per serving: 6.4 g (17%)

2½ cups chicken broth
1 pound red potatoes, peeled and cut into ½-inch pieces
1 cup chopped celery
¾ cup chopped scallion
1½ cups skim milk
½ cup evaporated skim milk
¼ cup all-purpose flour
¼ teaspoon black pepper
¼ teaspoon cayenne
2 tablespoons dry sherry
1½ cups peeled cooked shrimp
½ medium-sized red bell pepper, chopped
2 tablespoons chopped fresh parsley
½ teaspoon Worcestershire sauce
½ teaspoon paprika
¾ cup (3 ounces) grated reduced-fat sharp cheddar cheese
½ teaspoon salt

1. In a dutch oven, bring broth to a boil. Add potatoes, celery, and scallion, return to a boil, reduce heat, cover tightly, and simmer for 10 minutes or until potatoes are tender. Slowly stir in skim milk.

2. In a small bowl, whisk together evaporated milk and flour until smooth. Whisk evaporated milk mixture into pot. Mash about one-third of the potatoes into the soup. Add black pepper and cayenne and cook over medium heat until thickened. Stir in sherry, shrimp, bell pepper, parsley, Worcestershire sauce, and paprika.

3. Remove from heat, stir in cheese and salt, and stir until cheese is melted. Cover and let stand for at least 30 minutes to allow flavors to blend. Reheat, if necessary, over low heat.

STACKED TURKEY SANDWICHES, GREEN PEA SALAD, AND CRANBERRY SPRITZER

Serves 4

Total calories per serving: 350
Total fat per serving: 3.8 g (10%)

STACKED TURKEY SANDWICHES *(135 calories, 1 g fat per serving)*

¼ cup fat-free mayonnaise-style
  salad dressing
1 tablespoon plus 1 teaspoon
  Dijon mustard
8 slices light Italian bread
4 lettuce leaves
8 ½-ounce slices honey-roasted
  turkey
4 thin slices red onion
4 slices tomato
Alfalfa sprouts to taste
2 kosher pickles, split lengthwise

In a small bowl, combine salad dressing and mustard until well blended. Spread mixture on bread. Top each of four slices with one lettuce leaf, 1 ounce turkey, one slice onion, one slice tomato, and some alfalfa sprouts. Top with remaining slice of bread, cut, and serve with pickle.

GREEN PEA SALAD *(155 calories, 2.8 g fat per serving)*

½ cup fat-free mayonnaise-style
  salad dressing
⅓ cup finely chopped yellow
  onion
1 teaspoon sugar
½ teaspoon black pepper
24 small green olives stuffed with
  pimientos, sliced
2 10-ounce packages frozen green
  peas, steam cooked

Combine salad dressing, onion, sugar, pepper, and olives. Blend thoroughly. Add peas. Toss gently but thoroughly to coat completely. Refrigerate for 1 hour.

(Continued on the next page)

CRANBERRY SPRITZER *(60 calories, 0 g fat per serving)*

1⅓ cups low-calorie cranberry
    juice drink
1 cup white or purple grape juice
1 teaspoon fresh lemon juice
1 teaspoon fresh lime juice
Ice cubes
1⅓ cups sparkling mineral water
4 slices lemon or lime for garnish

1. In a pitcher, combine juices. Stir to blend thoroughly. Chill.

2. At serving time, fill glasses with ice. Gently stir sparkling water into juice in pitcher, pour equal amounts over ice, garnish with lemon or lime slices, and serve immediately.

SUGAR-GLAZED CHICKEN AND ORANGE-CURRY SALAD WITH PEANUTS

Serves 4

Total calories per serving: 349
Total fat per serving: 6.8 g (18%)

¾ pound skinless, boneless chicken breast, cut into thin strips
⅓ cup low-sodium soy sauce
5 tablespoons plus 2 teaspoons dark brown sugar
2 teaspoons fresh lime juice
1 teaspoon hot red pepper flakes
1 tablespoon plus ½ teaspoon curry powder
½ teaspoon ground ginger
2 teaspoons dry mustard
1 cup fresh orange juice
2 teaspoons cornstarch
2 teaspoons cider vinegar
8 cups torn spinach leaves
½ cup thinly sliced red onion
½ cup thinly sliced red bell pepper
½ cup sliced water chestnuts
1 8-ounce can juice-packed pineapple chunks, well drained
Butter-flavored cooking spray
¼ cup (1¼ ounces) peanuts, toasted in broiler

1. Place chicken in a shallow glass baking dish or gallon-size zip-lock bag. Combine soy sauce, 4 tablespoons plus 1 teaspoon brown sugar, lime juice, red pepper flakes, ½ teaspoon curry powder, ginger, and 1 teaspoon dry mustard. Whisk together to blend well and pour over chicken; stir and refrigerate for 1–3 hours.

2. In a small saucepan, combine orange juice, cornstarch, vinegar, remaining 1 tablespoon plus 1 teaspoon brown sugar, remaining tablespoon curry powder, and remaining teaspoon dry mustard. Stir until cornstarch dissolves, then place over medium-high heat, bring to a boil, and continue boiling for 1 minute, stirring occasionally. Chill thoroughly.

3. At serving time, arrange 2 cups torn spinach on each of four dinner plates. Evenly divide onion, bell pepper, water chestnuts, and pineapple chunks over spinach. Set plates aside.

4. Liberally coat a large nonstick skillet with cooking spray and place over high heat for 1 minute. Add chicken and marinade to skillet and cook, stirring, for about 5 minutes or until all liquid is absorbed and a glaze appears. Place equal amounts of chicken in center of salads. Stir chilled orange-curry dressing. If too thick, stir in 1–2 teaspoons water, then drizzle ¼ cup dressing around outer edges of each salad. Top each with 1 tablespoon toasted peanuts. Serve immediately.

CANTALOUPE HALVES STUFFED WITH CURRIED CHICKEN SALAD

Serves 4

Total calories per serving: 345
Total fat per serving: 5 g (13%)

7 tablespoons fat-free
  mayonnaise-style salad dressing
1 tablespoon plus 1 teaspoon
  sugar
1 tablespoon plus 1 teaspoon
  fresh lemon juice
2 teaspoons low-sodium soy
  sauce
2 teaspoons curry powder
1 teaspoon dry mustard
½ teaspoon hot red pepper flakes
¼ teaspoon salt
⅛ teaspoon ground ginger
⅛ teaspoon ground nutmeg
4 cups chopped cooked white
  chicken meat
½ cup sliced water chestnuts,
  slivered
¼ cup chopped red bell pepper
¼ cup chopped scallion
2 5-inch cantaloupes, halved and
  seeded
Paprika for garnish

1. In a mixing bowl, combine salad dressing, sugar, lemon juice, soy sauce, curry, mustard, red pepper flakes, salt, ginger, and nutmeg. Blend thoroughly. Add chicken, water chestnuts, bell pepper, and scallion. Blend gently but thoroughly. Chill for 1 hour.
2. At serving time, place one-fourth of chicken mixture in each cantaloupe half, sprinkle with paprika, and serve.

CHICKEN WITH LIME CREOLE SAUCE IN TORTILLAS

Serves 4

Total calories per serving: 349
Total fat per serving: 7.8 g (20%)

5 tablespoons plus 1 teaspoon fat-free mayonnaise-style salad dressing
6 tablespoons nonfat sour cream
1 teaspoon grated lime zest
¼ cup fresh lime juice
2 teaspoons chili powder
½ teaspoon black pepper
⅛ teaspoon cayenne pepper
¼ teaspoon salt
12 drops Louisiana hot sauce or to taste
3 4-ounce skinless, boneless chicken breasts
Butter-flavored cooking spray
¼ teaspoon garlic powder
8 6-inch flour tortillas, warmed
2 cups shredded lettuce
1 large tomato, chopped
½ cup chopped red onion
½ cup chopped green bell pepper
16 medium-sized pitted black olives, quartered
Lime wedges for garnish

1. In a small nonaluminum bowl, combine salad dressing, sour cream, lime zest, juice, chili powder, ¼ teaspoon black pepper, cayenne, salt, and hot sauce. Blend thoroughly and chill for 1 hour.

2. Flatten chicken breasts to ¼-inch thickness. Liberally coat a large nonstick skillet with cooking spray and place over high heat until hot, about 1½–2 minutes. Add chicken, sprinkle with garlic powder and remaining ¼ teaspoon black pepper, and cook for 2 minutes. Turn and cook for 2 minutes longer or until no longer pink in center. Immediately remove from heat and cut into thin strips.

3. Spread 2 tablespoons chilled sauce evenly on each tortilla. Top each with equal amounts of chicken, lettuce, tomato, onion, bell pepper, and olives. Roll tortillas and serve immediately with lime wedges.

CHICKEN AND PEPPERONCINI SALAD WITH FETA AND FRESH CROUTONS

Serves 4

Total calories per serving: 350
Total fat per serving: 10.9 g (28%)

Dressing
¼ cup cider vinegar
1 tablespoon plus 1 teaspoon
  extra-virgin olive oil
2 tablespoons dry white wine
½ teaspoon salt
¼ teaspoon black pepper
2 cloves garlic, minced
½ teaspoon dry mustard
½ teaspoon dried oregano leaves
½ teaspoon Louisiana hot sauce
  or to taste

Salad
12 cups torn mixed green lettuce
  leaves
12 plum tomatoes, seeded and
  sliced thin lengthwise
8 water-packed canned artichoke
  hearts, drained and quartered
¼ cup thinly sliced red onion
8 pepperoncini, sliced thin
  crosswise
¼ cup chopped fresh parsley
1 cup (about 6 ounces) chopped
  cooked white chicken meat
1½ ounces feta cheese, crumbled
  (about ⅓ cup)

Croutons
Olive oil–flavored cooking spray
4 1-ounce slices Italian bread,
  cut into ¼-inch cubes
Garlic powder to taste

3 tablespoons freshly grated
  Parmesan cheese
Freshly ground black pepper
  (if desired)

1. Preheat oven to 350°F.
2. In a small jar, combine all dressing ingredients. Shake well and refrigerate until serving time.
3. Place mixed greens in a large salad bowl. Decoratively arrange all other salad ingredients on top. Refrigerate until serving time.
4. Coat a nonstick baking sheet with cooking spray. Place bread cubes on sheet in a single layer, liberally spray cooking spray over bread cubes, and sprinkle with garlic powder. Bake for 13–15 minutes or until browned.
5. At serving time, shake salad dressing well and pour over salad. Toss gently but thoroughly to coat lettuce leaves. Add Parmesan and toss lightly. Place equal amounts on 4 dinner plates, top with croutons, and sprinkle with pepper.

Variation: Replace chicken with 1 cup chilled cooked bowtie pasta (338 calories, 9.9 g fat (26%) per serving).

LOUISIANA BLACKENED CHICKEN SALAD WITH TOASTED CAJUN BREAD

Serves 4

Total calories per serving: 339
Total fat per serving: 8.4 g (22%)

LOUISIANA BLACKENED CHICKEN SALAD (244 calories, 7.4 g fat per serving)

Salad

¼ cup red wine vinegar
1 tablespoon extra-virgin olive oil
1 2-ounce jar chopped pimiento
2 cloves garlic, minced
2 tablespoons drained capers
1 tablespoon plus 2 teaspoons
   Louisiana hot sauce or to taste
¼ teaspoon salt
⅛ teaspoon black pepper
½ pound mushrooms, sliced
4 scallions, chopped
24 cherry tomatoes
10 cups torn mixed salad greens

Chicken

¾ pound skinless, boneless
   chicken breasts
¼ teaspoon cayenne pepper
⅛ teaspoon black pepper
¼ teaspoon salt
⅛ teaspoon ground cumin
¼ teaspoon paprika
Cooking spray

Freshly ground black pepper to
   taste

1. In a salad bowl, combine vinegar, oil, pimiento, garlic, capers, hot sauce, salt, and pepper. Whisk until well blended. Add mushrooms and scallions. Toss to coat thoroughly. Refrigerate for 30 minutes.

2. Flatten chicken breasts to ¼-inch thickness. In a small bowl, combine cayenne, black pepper, salt, cumin, and paprika. Mix thoroughly. Sprinkle evenly over both sides of chicken pieces and rub into meat.

3. Liberally coat a large skillet, preferably cast iron, with cooking spray and place over high heat until very hot, about 2 minutes. Be sure your kitchen is well ventilated. Place chicken pieces in hot skillet and cook for 2 minutes. Turn and cook for 1½–2 minutes longer or until no longer pink in center. Cut into thin strips.

4. Toss tomatoes and mixed greens with dressing in salad bowl. Place equal amounts on each of four dinner plates. Top each with equal amounts of chicken. Sprinkle freshly ground black pepper over all and serve immediately.

(Continued on the next page)

TOASTED CAJUN BREAD *(95 calories, 1 g fat per serving)*

4 1-ounce slices Italian bread
2 teaspoons light margarine,
    softened
Cajun or Creole seasoning to
    taste

1. Preheat broiler.
2. Spread ½ teaspoon margarine onto each slice of bread. Sprinkle seasoning on each slice. Set slices on broiler rack and broil for 1–2 minutes, or until bread is lightly toasted. Serve one slice with each serving of salad.

QUICK ITALIAN BEEF PIZZA BREAD AND SIMPLE TOSSED SALAD WITH PARMESAN

Serves 4

Total calories per serving: 348
Total fat per serving: 8.2 g (21%)

QUICK ITALIAN BEEF PIZZA BREAD *(308 calories, 7.7 g fat per serving)*

½ pound lean ground round
Cooking spray
2 cloves garlic, minced
1 cup sliced fresh mushrooms
½ cup chopped yellow onion
⅓ cup chopped green bell pepper
2 tablespoons chopped fresh
　parsley
8 ounces Italian bread, split
　length-wise
½ cup bottled pizza sauce
½ teaspoon dried basil leaves
½ teaspoon dried oregano leaves
1 cup (4 ounces) grated part-skim
　mozzarella cheese
4 teaspoons freshly grated
　Parmesan cheese
Hot red pepper flakes (if desired)

1. Preheat oven to 475°F.
2. Place a large nonstick skillet over medium-high heat, add ground round, and cook until brown. Place on paper towels and blot well.
3. Wipe skillet with paper towels, coat with cooking spray, and place over medium-high heat. Add garlic, mushrooms, onion, and bell pepper. Cook for 4 minutes or until vegetables are limp. Stir in parsley and set aside. Cut bread in half crosswise to form 4 pieces.
4. Spoon 2 tablespoons pizza sauce over each slice of bread. Sprinkle each with ⅛ teaspoon basil, ⅛ teaspoon oregano, one-fourth of the cooked beef, and one-fourth of the vegetable mixture. Top each with ¼ cup mozzarella cheese. Place on a foil-lined oven rack and bake for 4–5 minutes or until cheese has melted. Sprinkle each with 1 teaspoon Parmesan cheese and with hot red pepper flakes if desired.

SIMPLE TOSSED SALAD WITH PARMESAN *(40 calories, 0.5 g fat per serving)*

4 cups torn mixed lettuce leaves
8 cherry tomatoes, halved
½ cup bottled fat-free Italian
　salad dressing
4 teaspoons grated Parmesan

Place 1 cup lettuce and four tomato halves onto each of four plates. Top each with 2 tablespoons dressing and 1 teaspoon Parmesan.

ROAST BEEF SALAD WITH BLUE CHEESE IN PITAS AND SLICED FRESH APPLES

Serves 4

Total calories per serving: 346
Total fat per serving: 6.5 g (17%)

ROAST BEEF SALAD WITH BLUE CHEESE IN PITAS *(306 calories, 6.2 g fat per serving)*

½ cup fat-free mayonnaise-style
  salad dressing
2 tablespoons plus 2 teaspoons
  Dijon mustard
2 teaspoons prepared horseradish
4 loaves pita, halved to make
  pockets
16 ½-ounce slices lean cooked
  deli roast beef
2 cups shredded lettuce
½ cup chopped tomato
½ cup chopped cucumber,
  peeled if desired
½ cup alfalfa sprouts
¼ cup (2 ounces) crumbled blue
  cheese

In a small bowl, combine salad dressing, mustard, and horseradish; mix well and set aside. Fill each pita half with two slices beef, 1 tablespoon plus 1 teaspoon sauce, ¼ cup lettuce, 1 tablespoon tomato, 1 tablespoon cucumber, and 1 tablespoon alfalfa sprouts. Top with 1½ teaspoons blue cheese.

SLICED FRESH APPLES *(40 calories, 0.3 g fat per serving)*

2 medium-sized apples (any
  variety)

Peel apples, if desired. Cut each into eight wedges. Serve four wedges on each of four small plates.

HAMBURGERS ON TOASTED BUNS WITH PICKLE SPEARS

Serves 4

Total calories per serving: 344
Total fat per serving: 8 g (21%)

1 pound lean ground round
¼ cup finely chopped yellow
  onion
2 cloves garlic, minced
1 tablespoon plus 1 teaspoon
  Dijon mustard
Cooking spray
1 tablespoon low-sodium soy
  sauce
1 tablespoon Worcestershire
  sauce
⅛ teaspoon barbecue smoke
  seasoning
Paprika to taste
Black pepper to taste
4 hamburger buns, toasted
4 lettuce leaves
4 slices tomato
4 thin slices onion
¼ cup fat-free mayonnaise-style
  salad dressing
4 teaspoons mustard
4 teaspoons ketchup
4 1-ounce dill pickles, quartered
  lengthwise

1. Preheat the broiler.
2. Combine ground round, onion, garlic, and Dijon mustard. Mix until just blended; do not overmix. Shape into four patties. Coat broiler rack and broiler pan with cooking spray.
3. Place patties on rack no less than 2–3 inches from heat source. Combine soy sauce, Worcestershire, and smoke seasoning and set aside. Broil beef for 3 minutes. Turn, spoon soy sauce mixture evenly over burgers, and sprinkle with paprika and liberally with black pepper. Broil for 3–3½ minutes longer or until cooked to taste. Place on toasted buns and pile each with lettuce, tomato, onion, 1 tablespoon salad dressing, 1 teaspoon mustard, and 1 teaspoon ketchup. Serve each burger with four pickle spears.

WILD RICE–SAUSAGE CHOWDER AND FRESH TOMATO SLICES

Serves 4

Total calories per serving: 346
Total fat per serving: 7.6 g (20%)

WILD RICE–SAUSAGE CHOWDER *(330 calories, 7.6 g fat per serving)*

1 6-ounce box Uncle Ben's Long Grain & Wild Rice and seasoning packet
Cooking spray
½ pound bulk turkey sausage
1 16-ounce can chicken broth
1 cup chopped celery
1 cup chopped onion
½ cup chopped red or green bell pepper
½ cup chopped carrot
3 tablespoons chopped fresh parsley
½ teaspoon dried oregano leaves
⅛ teaspoon black pepper
⅛ teaspoon cayenne pepper
2 cups skim milk
2 tablespoons plus 2 teaspoons all-purpose flour
1 tablespoon Worcestershire sauce
Paprika for garnish

1. Cook rice according to package directions, omitting salt and margarine. Meanwhile, coat a dutch oven, preferably cast iron, with cooking spray and place over medium-high heat. Add sausage, breaking up with a knife and fork, and cook until brown. Set aside on paper towels.

2. Add broth to dutch oven and bring to a boil. Add celery, onion, bell pepper, and carrots, return to a boil, reduce heat, cover tightly, and simmer for 4 minutes or until crisp-tender. Add parsley, oregano, black pepper, cayenne, and 2 cups of the cooked rice (reserve remaining rice for another use).

3. In a small container, combine ½ cup of the milk and the flour; whisk until smooth. Add to dutch oven with remaining milk, sausage, and Worcestershire sauce. Bring to a boil, immediately reduce heat, stir, cover tightly, and simmer for 10 minutes or until thickened. Remove from heat, sprinkle with paprika, and let stand, covered, for 10 minutes to blend flavors.

FRESH TOMATO SLICES *(16 calories, 0 g fat per serving)*

2 medium-sized tomatoes

Thinly slice tomatoes. Serve one-fourth of tomato slices on each of four small plates.

HEARTY SAUSAGE AND PASTA STEW AND MIXED GREENS WITH CREAMY LEMON GARLIC DRESSING

Serves 4

Total calories per serving: 349
Total fat per serving: 10.3 g (27%)

HEARTY SAUSAGE AND PASTA STEW (307 calories, 8.1 g fat per serving)

Cooking spray
10 ounces turkey sausage links, cut into ⅛-inch rounds
2 cups chopped yellow onion
4 cloves garlic, minced
1½ cups sliced zucchini
1 medium-sized green bell pepper, chopped
1 10-ounce can condensed beef broth
1 16-ounce can chicken broth
1 cup dry red wine
½ cup water
1 8-ounce can tomato sauce
1 16-ounce can peeled whole tomatoes, chopped, undrained
1 teaspoon dried basil leaves
1 teaspoon dried oregano leaves
¼ teaspoon black pepper
¼ cup chopped fresh parsley
2 teaspoons Worcestershire sauce
½ teaspoon sugar
2 cups cooked penne, no butter, margarine, or oil used in cooking

1. Coat a dutch oven, preferably cast iron, with cooking spray and place over medium-high heat 1 minute. Add sausage, brown lightly, and set aside.
2. Add onion and garlic to dutch oven and cook, stirring occasionally, for 4 minutes. Add zucchini, bell pepper, beef broth, chicken broth, wine, water, tomato sauce, tomatoes and their liquid, basil, oregano, and black pepper. Bring to a boil, reduce heat, cover tightly, and simmer for 20 minutes. Stir in parsley, Worcestershire sauce, sugar, pasta, and reserved sausage. Remove from heat and let stand, covered, for 10 minutes. Flavor is enhanced if refrigerated overnight.

(Continued on the next page)

MIXED GREENS WITH CREAMY LEMON GARLIC DRESSING
(42 calories, 2.2 g fat per serving)

Dressing
1 cup plain nonfat yogurt
2 tablespoons fresh lemon juice
1 tablespoon plus 1½ teaspoons
    extra-virgin olive oil
2 tablespoons plus 1½ teaspoons
    Dijon mustard
1 clove garlic, minced
¼ teaspoon dried oregano leaves
¼ teaspoon salt
¼ teaspoon black pepper

Salad
4 cups mixed torn salad greens
1 cup thinly sliced cucumber,
    peeled if desired
¼ cup chopped red onion
Freshly ground black pepper to
    taste

1. Combine all dressing ingredients in a food processor and blend until smooth. Refrigerate until serving time.

2. Place greens, cucumber, and onion in a salad bowl. Toss with ½ cup dressing and sprinkle with freshly ground pepper. Place one-fourth of salad on each of four plates and serve. Remaining dressing may be refrigerated for up to two weeks, but not past the expiration date of the yogurt.

HAM, TOMATO, AND SPROUT SANDWICHES, POTATO SALAD, AND ORANGE FRESHER

Serves 4

Total calories per serving: 343
Total fat per serving: 3.4 g (9%)

HAM, TOMATO, AND SPROUT SANDWICHES (149 calories, 3.2 g fat)

8 slices light bread
8 ½-ounce slices lean ham
4 slices tomato
4 rings green or red bell pepper
¼ cup chopped scallion
16 fresh spinach leaves, washed
2 cups alfalfa or bean sprouts
Black pepper to taste
¼ cup fat-free mayonnaise-style
   salad dressing
1 tablespoon plus 1 teaspoon
   Dijon mustard

1. On each of four slices bread, place two slices ham, one slice tomato, one ring bell pepper, 1 tablespoon scallion, four spinach leaves, and ½ cup sprouts. Sprinkle with pepper.

2. Mix salad dressing and mustard together. Spread one-fourth of the mixture on each of the remaining four slices bread. Place bread on top and serve.

POTATO SALAD (125 calories, 0.2 g fat per serving)

1 quart water
1 pound red potatoes, peeled and
   cut into ½-inch pieces (about 3
   cups)
½ cup fat-free mayonnaise-style
   salad dressing
2 tablespoons skim milk
2 teaspoons cider vinegar
2 teaspoons mustard
½ teaspoon salt
⅛ teaspoon black pepper
½ cup chopped celery
½ cup chopped dill pickle
½ cup chopped green bell pepper
½ cup chopped yellow onion
Paprika for garnish

1. In a 2-quart saucepan, bring water to a boil. Add potatoes, return to a boil, reduce heat, and simmer, uncovered, for 7 minutes or until tender. Remove from heat and let stand for 1 minute. Drain well and cool completely.

2. In a mixing bowl, combine remaining ingredients except paprika; mix well. Add cooled potatoes and toss gently but thoroughly to coat completely. Sprinkle with paprika and chill for at least 3 hours to allow potatoes to absorb flavors.

(Continued on the next page)

ORANGE FRESHER *(69 calories, 0 g fat per serving)*

1⅓ cups fresh orange juice
1 cup white grape juice
Ice cubes
1 cup diet lemon-lime soda

In a pitcher, combine orange juice and white grape juice. Stir well and chill. At serving time, fill tall glasses with ice, add soda to juice in pitcher, and stir gently but thoroughly. Pour equal amounts over ice and serve immediately.

FIRESIDE WHITE BEAN AND SAUSAGE SOUP WITH SIMPLE SPICED ITALIAN SALAD

Serves 4

Total calories per serving: 348
Total fat per serving: 9.5 g (25%)

FIRESIDE WHITE BEAN AND SAUSAGE SOUP (328 calories, 9.5 g fat per serving)

¾ pound turkey sausage links, cut into ⅛-inch rounds
2 cups chopped yellow onion
1 16-ounce can chicken broth
¼ cup water
2 bay leaves
1 teaspoon dried thyme leaves
¼ teaspoon black pepper
¼ teaspoon cayenne pepper
2 16-ounce cans butter beans, well rinsed and drained
1 tablespoon plus 1 teaspoon ketchup

1. Place a dutch oven, preferably cast iron, over medium heat, add sausage, and cook until *just* beginning to brown. Add onion and cook for 6–8 minutes or until transparent.

2. Add broth, water, bay leaves, thyme, black pepper, and cayenne, scraping bottom and sides. Bring to a boil, reduce heat, cover tightly, and simmer for 5 minutes.

3. Add beans, reduce heat to a very low simmer, and cook for 4 minutes longer, uncovered. Remove from heat, gently stir in ketchup, cover tightly, and let stand for 20 minutes.

4. Remove bay leaves and serve.

SIMPLE SPICED ITALIAN SALAD (20 calories, 0 g fat per serving)

4 cups torn mixed salad greens
¼ cup finely chopped red onion
½ cup bottled fat-free Italian dressing
Louisiana hot sauce to taste

Toss together ingredients. Serve one-fourth of salad on each of four plates.

ROLLED HAM WITH CREAM CHEESE
AND SWEET RED POPPY FRUIT–LETTUCE PLATTER

Serves 4

Total calories per serving: 341
Total fat per serving: 8 g (21%)

ROLLED HAM WITH CREAM CHEESE *(105 calories, 2.8 g fat per serving)*

½ cup fat-free cream cheese
3 tablespoons chopped scallion
3 tablespoons chopped fresh
  parsley
1 clove garlic, minced
¼ teaspoon black pepper
8 1-ounce slices lean ham
32 toothpicks

In a food processor, combine cream cheese, scallion, parsley, garlic, and pepper. Process until well blended. Spread evenly over ham slices. Roll up in jelly roll fashion, cut each roll into fourths, secure with toothpicks, and chill thoroughly.

SWEET RED POPPY FRUIT–LETTUCE PLATTER *(236 calories, 5.2 g fat per serving)*

Dressing
1 cup water
1 tablespoon plus 1 teaspoon
  cornstarch
½ cup sugar
6 tablespoons cider vinegar
2 tablespoons vegetable oil
1 tablespoon paprika
1 tablespoon poppy seeds
½ teaspoon dry mustard
¼ teaspoon salt

1. In a small saucepan, combine water and cornstarch and stir until cornstarch dissolves. Bring to a boil, stirring frequently, and boil for 1 minute longer. Remove from heat and stir in remaining dressing ingredients. Chill thoroughly.

2. On each of four dinner plates, place 3 cups lettuce, 3 tablespoons scallion, and ¼ cup each oranges, pineapple, strawberries, grapes, watermelon, and honeydew on top of lettuce. Drizzle ¼ cup of the dressing over each salad and serve immediately.

Salad
12 cups torn mixed greens such
  as spinach, romaine, and
  escarole
¾ cup chopped scallion
1 cup well-drained juice-packed
  canned mandarin oranges

1 cup well-drained juice-packed
  pineapple chunks
1 cup sliced strawberries
1 cup seedless red or green grapes
1 cup watermelon cubes
1 cup honeydew cubes

STUFFED POTATOES WITH VEGETABLES, CHEESE, AND BACON, SOUR CREAM–SCALLION SALAD, AND SLICED FRESH APPLES

Serves 4

Total calories per serving: 346
Total fat per serving: 6.9 g (18%)

STUFFED POTATOES WITH VEGETABLES, CHEESE, AND BACON
(259 calories, 6.2 g fat per serving)

4 ½-pound white potatoes,
   wrapped in foil
Butter-flavored cooking spray
2 cloves garlic, minced
1 cup chopped yellow onion
1 cup chopped green bell pepper
6 ounces (about 2 cups)
   mushrooms, quartered
1 cup cooked green beans
2 tablespoons chopped fresh
   parsley
1 teaspoon Worcestershire sauce
½ cup (2 ounces) grated reduced-
   fat sharp cheddar cheese
4 slices lower-sodium bacon,
   cooked, blotted dry, and
   crumbled
Freshly ground black pepper to
   taste

1. Preheat oven to 350°F.
2. Place potatoes in oven and bake for 1 hour.
3. While potatoes are baking, coat a large nonstick skillet with cooking spray and place over medium-high heat for 1 minute. Add garlic, onion, bell pepper, and mushrooms. Cook for 8 minutes. Stir in green beans, parsley, and Worcestershire sauce and cook for 3 minutes longer.
4. When potatoes are done, split them in half lengthwise and fluff potatoes with a fork, being careful not to tear skins. Fill with equal amounts of vegetables and top with cheese. Place back in oven to melt, about 3 minutes. Top each with one-fourth of the bacon. Sprinkle pepper over all and serve.

(Continued on the next page)

SOUR CREAM–SCALLION SALAD *(47 calories, 0.4 g fat per serving)*

Dressing
¼ cup nonfat sour cream
¼ cup nonfat buttermilk
1 teaspoon fresh lemon juice
1 teaspoon prepared horseradish
¼ teaspoon salt
¼ teaspoon black pepper
2 tablespoons chopped scallion

Salad
4 cups torn romaine lettuce
   leaves
½ cup peeled and sliced
   cucumber
8 cherry tomatoes

1. In a small mixing bowl, combine sour cream, buttermilk, lemon juice, horseradish, salt, and pepper. Whisk to blend thoroughly. Stir in scallion and chill until serving time.

2. At serving time, place on each salad plate 1 cup torn lettuce, one-fourth of the cucumber slices, and two tomatoes. Spoon 2 tablespoons dressing over each serving. Serve immediately.

SLICED FRESH APPLES *(40 calories, 0.3 g fat per serving)*

**2 medium-sized apples (any
   variety)**

Peel apples, if desired. Cut each into eight wedges. Serve four wedges on each of four small plates.

HAM SLICES WITH SWEET CURRY, FRUIT, AND RICE SALAD AND MELBA ROUNDS WITH CREAM CHEESE

Serves 4

Total calories per serving: 348
Total fat per serving: 3.8 g (10%)

HAM SLICES WITH SWEET CURRY, FRUIT, AND RICE SALAD
(283 calories, 3 g fat per serving)

⅓ cup fat-free mayonnaise-style salad dressing
⅓ cup plain nonfat yogurt
1 tablespoon plus 1 teaspoon dark brown sugar
2 teaspoons curry powder
½ teaspoon ground ginger
½ teaspoon dry mustard
¼ teaspoon salt
8 1-ounce lean ham slices
4 lettuce leaves
½ cup drained juice-packed crushed pineapple
½ cup drained juice-packed mandarin oranges
½ cup seedless red or green grape halves
¼ cup chopped scallion
¼ cup chopped red or green bell pepper
3 cups cold cooked white rice, no butter, margarine, or oil used in cooking

1. In a small bowl, combine salad dressing, yogurt, brown sugar, curry powder, ginger, mustard, and salt. Blend thoroughly and set aside.

2. Arrange two ham slices and a lettuce leaf on each of four plates. Combine pineapple, oranges, grapes, scallion, bell pepper, rice, and mayonnaise mixture. Toss well to blend. Spoon equal amounts on lettuce leaves and serve immediately.

MELBA ROUNDS WITH CREAM CHEESE *(65 calories, 0.8 g fat)*

¼ cup fat-free cream cheese
12 melba rounds
Ground cinnamon to taste

Spread 1 teaspoon cream cheese onto each round. Sprinkle with cinnamon. Serve 3 rounds on each of four small plates.

FRESH GARDEN RAVIOLI AND MOZZARELLA SOUP
WITH ASPARAGUS SPEAR SALAD

Serves 4

Total calories per serving: 344
Total fat per serving: 11.3 g (30%)

FRESH GARDEN RAVIOLI AND MOZZARELLA SOUP *(277 calories, 8.5 g fat per serving)*

2 16-ounce cans chicken broth
1 9-ounce package refrigerated
   Contadina Light Garden
   Vegetable Ravioli
2 cloves garlic, minced
1 tablespoon minced fresh
   parsley
¼ teaspoon dried basil leaves
⅛ teaspoon black pepper
1 cup (¼ pound) grated part-skim
   mozzarella cheese
4 teaspoons freshly grated
   Parmesan cheese

In a medium-sized saucepan, bring broth to a boil. Add ravioli, garlic, parsley, basil, and black pepper. Return to a boil, reduce heat, and simmer, uncovered, for 8 minutes or until done, gently separating ravioli with a fork midway through cooking. Remove from heat, cover, and let stand for 5 minutes to blend flavors. Spoon equal amounts of soup into bowls and sprinkle ¼ cup grated mozzarella and 1 teaspoon grated Parmesan on top of each.

ASPARAGUS SPEAR SALAD *(67 calories, 2.8 g fat per serving)*

Salad
1 pound fresh asparagus, ends
   trimmed

Creamy Dijon Dressing
½ cup plain nonfat yogurt
2½ teaspoon extra-virgin olive oil
1 tablespoon plus 1 teaspoon
   Dijon mustard
1 clove garlic, minced
½ teaspoon salt
¼ teaspoon black pepper
1 tablespoon plus 1 teaspoon
   freshly grated Parmesan cheese

1. Lightly steam asparagus until tender but crisp. Refrigerate for 15–20 minutes.
2. Combine all dressing ingredients in a blender and blend until smooth. Chill. Makes about ⅔ cup.
3. Place one-fourth of the spears on each of four small plates. Drizzle 2 tablespoons dressing over each serving. Remaining dressing may be refrigerated for up to two weeks, but not past the expiration date of the yogurt.

BEAN AND CHEESE TOSTADAS, SIMPLE PEPPERED SALAD, AND LIMEADE

Serves 4

Total calories per serving: 342
Total fat per serving: 7.6 g (20%)

BEAN AND CHEESE TOSTADAS *(232 calories, 7.6 g fat per serving)*

¾ cup well-rinsed and drained canned red kidney beans

1 medium-sized tomato, seeded and chopped

¼ cup drained canned green chilies

¼ cup chopped scallion

2 tablespoons chopped fresh cilantro leaves

1 teaspoon chili powder

4 6-inch corn tortillas

1 cup (¼ pound) grated reduced-fat sharp cheddar cheese

¼ cup nonfat sour cream

12 medium-sized pitted black olives, quartered

1. Preheat the broiler.
2. In a mixing bowl, combine beans, tomato, chilies, scallion, cilantro, and chili powder. Mix well and set aside. Place two tortillas on each of two baking sheets. Top each tortilla with one-fourth of the bean mixture and sprinkle with ¼ cup cheese. Place one baking sheet under broiler no less than 5 inches from heat source and broil for 2–3 minutes or until cheese melts and edges of tortilla begin to curl up and take on a "dish" appearance. Repeat with remaining two tortillas. Top each with 1 tablespoon sour cream and one-fourth of the olives. Serve immediately.

SIMPLE PEPPERED SALAD *(51 calories, 0 g fat per serving)*

3 cups torn mixed salad greens

1 cup sliced cucumber, peeled if desired

¼ cup chopped scallion

½ cup bottled fat-free ranch dressing

Freshly ground black pepper to taste

Place ¾ cup salad greens in each of four salad bowls. Top with ¼ cup cucumber and 1 tablespoon scallion. Spoon 2 tablespoons dressing over each and *liberally* sprinkle with black pepper.

(Continued on the next page)

LIMEADE (59 calories, 0 g fat per serving)

4 medium-sized fresh limes
¼ cup sugar
4 packets (1⅓ teaspoons) Equal
3 cups water
Ice cubes

1. Grate ½ teaspoon lime zest from one of the limes, being careful not to grate the bitter white area. Place zest in a blender. Roll limes on a hard surface to soften thoroughly. Cut each in half and squeeze all the juice into blender. Add sugar, Equal, and water and blend thoroughly until sugar dissolves.

2. Immediately fill four glasses with ice and pour equal amounts limeade over ice. Serve.

HOT OPEN-FACED CHEESE SANDWICHES AND RASPBERRY-WINE VINAIGRETTE SALAD

Serves 4

Total calories per serving: 342
Total fat per serving: 9.7 g (26%)

HOT OPEN-FACED CHEESE SANDWICHES (207 calories, 3.6 g fat per serving)

¼ cup (1 ounce) grated reduced-fat sharp cheddar cheese
¼ cup (1 ounce) grated part-skim mozzarella cheese
6 tablespoons fat-free mayonnaise-style salad dressing
¼ teaspoon curry powder
2 tablespoons finely chopped onion
1 tablespoon evaporated skim milk
Dash cayenne pepper
½ pound Italian bread, split lengthwise and cut into 4 pieces
Paprika for garnish

1. Combine all ingredients except bread and paprika in a mixing bowl. Blend thoroughly. Refrigerate overnight or for at least 2 hours.
2. Preheat the broiler. Spread cheese mixture evenly over bread slices, then sprinkle with paprika. Place on broiler pan no less than 5 inches from heat source. Broil for 3 minutes or until cheese is beginning to brown. Serve immediately.

(Continued on the next page)

RASPBERRY-WINE VINAIGRETTE SALAD *(135 calories, 6.1 g fat per serving)*

Dressing
¼ cup raspberry vinegar
3 tablespoons semisweet white
   wine
2 tablespoons vegetable oil
1 tablespoon sugar
¼ teaspoon dry mustard
¼ teaspoon salt
⅛ teaspoon black pepper

Salad
4 cups mixed greens such as
   Boston lettuce, Bibb lettuce,
   romaine lettuce, and endive
¼ cup chopped red onion
2 cups quartered strawberries
2 medium-sized navel oranges,
   sectioned
Freshly ground pepper to taste
   (if desired)

1. Mix dressing ingredients and refrigerate until serving time.

2. Place salad greens, onion, strawberries, and orange sections in a decorative bowl. Toss gently but thoroughly with ½ cup salad dressing (you'll have a little left over). Top with freshly ground black pepper if desired, and serve immediately.

JALAPENO-CHEESE CORN BREAD SQUARES WITH SALSA AND SLICED CUCUMBERS WITH SOUR CREAM DRESSING

Serves 4

Total calories per serving: 347
Total fat per serving: 11.1 g (29%)

JALAPENO-CHEESE CORN BREAD SQUARES WITH SALSA
(321 calories, 11 g fat per serving)

¼ cup egg substitute
1 cup self-rising yellow cornmeal mix
1 cup frozen corn kernels, thawed
¾ cup skim milk
1 tablespoon plus 2 teaspoons vegetable oil
¾ cup (3 ounces) grated reduced-fat sharp cheddar cheese
2 bottled jalapeño peppers, well drained and chopped (if desired)
Cooking spray
¾ cup bottled picante sauce
2 medium-sized tomatoes
¼ cup chopped red onion
1 tablespoon chopped fresh cilantro leaves (if desired)

1. Preheat oven to 450°F.

2. In a mixing bowl, combine egg substitute, cornmeal mix, corn kernels, milk, oil, cheese, and peppers. Stir until *just* blended. Place a nonstick 8-inch square baking pan in the hot oven for 3 minutes, remove from oven, immediately coat pan with cooking spray, pour batter into pan, and bake for 20 minutes.

3. Meanwhile, combine picante sauce, tomatoes, onion, and cilantro if desired and set aside.

4. When bread is done, immediately slice into four pieces, place on dinner plates, and top each with one-fourth of the tomato mixture. Serve immediately.

(Continued on the next page)

SLICED CUCUMBERS WITH SOUR CREAM DRESSING *(26 calories, 0.1 g fat per serving)*

Dressing

1 cup nonfat buttermilk

¼ cup fat-free mayonnaise-style salad dressing

¼ cup nonfat sour cream

1 tablespoon grated onion

¼ teaspoon garlic powder

¼ teaspoon black pepper

¼ teaspoon salt

Salad

3 cups peeled and sliced cucumber

Freshly ground black pepper to taste

1. In a mixing bowl, combine all dressing ingredients and whisk until well blended. Chill until serving time.

2. Arrange ¾ cup cucumber slices decoratively on each of four salad plates, spoon 2 tablespoons dressing over each salad and top with freshly ground black pepper. Remaining dressing may be refrigerated for up to one week, but not past expiration date of buttermilk, salad dressing, or sour cream.

EGG SALAD SANDWICHES, SLICED FRESH APPLES AND CHILLED GAZPACHO WITH FRESH CILANTRO

Serves 4

Total calories per serving: 304
Total fat per serving: 6.3 g (19%)

EGG SALAD SANDWICHES *(202 calories, 5.6 g fat per serving)*

¼ cup fat-free mayonnaise-style
  salad dressing
2 tablespoons plus 2 teaspoons
  sweet pickle relish
2 tablespoons plus 2 teaspoons
  finely chopped onion
¾ cup thinly sliced celery
⅛ teaspoon black pepper
4 large hard-cooked eggs,
  chopped
8 slices light bread, toasted if
  desired
4 slices tomato
4 lettuce leaves

1. In a mixing bowl, combine salad dressing, relish, onion, celery, and pepper. Mix well. Add chopped eggs and toss gently but thoroughly to blend completely. Chill until serving time.

2. Spread equal amounts of egg salad on four slices of bread, top each with a tomato slice and a lettuce leaf, and add remaining slice of bread. Serve immediately.

SLICED FRESH APPLES *(40 calories, 0.3 g fat per serving)*

2 medium-sized apples (any
  variety)

Peel apples, if desired. Cut each into eight wedges. Serve four wedges on each of four small plates.

(Continued on the next page)

CHILLED GAZPACHO WITH FRESH CILANTRO *(62 calories, 0.4 g fat per serving)*

3 cups tomato juice
1 cup peeled and chopped
   cucumber
2 medium-sized tomatoes,
   chopped
¼ cup finely chopped green bell
   pepper
¼ cup finely chopped yellow
   onion
⅓ cup chopped fresh cilantro
   leaves
2 tablespoons chopped radish
1 clove garlic, minced
2 tablespoons fresh lime juice
2 teaspoons Worcestershire sauce
¼ teaspoon sugar
Black pepper to taste
Louisiana hot sauce to taste

Combine all ingredients in a mixing bowl and chill for 1 hour.

WINTER VEGETABLE SOUP, GARLIC ITALIAN BREAD, AND CINNAMON-DUSTED APPLE SLICES

Serves 4

Total calories per serving: 350
Total fat per serving: 6.4 g (16%)

WINTER VEGETABLE SOUP *(173 calories, 3.7 g fat per serving)*

1 10-ounce can beef broth
1 14½-ounce can vegetable broth
1½ cups water
2 cups chopped green cabbage
½ pound red potatoes, peeled and diced
½ cup chopped celery
¼ cup chopped green bell pepper
1 cup diced cooked green beans
1 medium-sized tomato, seeded and chopped
3 tablespoons ketchup
1 bay leaf
½ teaspoon dried oregano leaves
½ teaspoon Worcestershire sauce
⅛ teaspoon black pepper
2 tablespoons chopped fresh parsley
1 tablespoon extra-virgin olive oil

In a dutch oven, preferably cast iron, bring beef broth, vegetable broth, and water to a boil. Add remaining ingredients except 1 tablespoon of the parsley and the oil. Return to a boil, reduce heat, cover tightly, and simmer for 15 minutes. Stir in oil and remaining tablespoon of parsley. Cover, remove from heat, and let stand for 10 minutes longer to blend flavors.

GARLIC ITALIAN BREAD *(96 calories, 2.2 g fat per serving)*

1 tablespoon plus 1 teaspoon light margarine, softened
1 clove garlic, minced
¼ pound Italian bread, split lengthwise
2 teaspoons freshly grated Parmesan cheese
1 tablespoon plus 1 teaspoon finely chopped fresh parsley

1. Preheat the broiler.
2. In a small container, combine margarine and garlic and blend thoroughly. Spread margarine mixture evenly on bread, sprinkle with Parmesan cheese, and top with parsley. Place on a foil-lined oven rack no less than 5 inches from heat source and broil for 1–2 minutes or until edges begin to brown and margarine mixture has melted. Cut bread into eight pieces and serve immediately (allow two pieces per serving).

(Continued on the next page)

CINNAMON-DUSTED APPLE SLICES *(81 calories, 0.5 g fat per serving)*

4 medium-sized apples (any variety)
Ground cinnamon to taste

Peel apples, if desired. Cut each apple into eighths, discarding core. Place eight slices on each of four small plates, lightly sprinkle with cinnamon, and serve.

MEDITERRANEAN COUSCOUS SALAD WITH FRESH LIMES, CUCUMBERS, AND TOMATOES

Serves 4

Total calories per serving: 345
Total fat per serving: 9.9 g (26%)

4 cups chilled cooked couscous,
   no butter, margarine, or oil
   used in cooking
5 medium-sized tomatoes
¼ cup finely chopped yellow
   onion
3 tablespoons chopped fresh
   parsley
¼ cup red wine vinegar
3 tablespoons fresh lime juice
2 cloves garlic, minced
½ teaspoon dried oregano leaves
½ teaspoon dry mustard
½ teaspoon salt
¼ teaspoon black pepper
1 tablespoon extra-virgin olive oil
⅓ cup freshly grated Parmesan
   cheese
2 tablespoons (1 ounce)
   crumbled feta cheese
12 Kalamata olives, pitted and
   quartered
4 lettuce leaves
1 medium-sized cucumber
Fresh lime wedges for garnish
Freshly ground black pepper to
   taste

1. Place chilled couscous in a mixing bowl. Seed and chop two of the tomatoes and add to couscous along with onion and parsley. In a small container, combine vinegar, lime juice, garlic, oregano, dry mustard, salt, and pepper. Mix thoroughly and pour over couscous mixture. Toss well and refrigerate for 2 hours.

2. Add oil and toss well. Add Parmesan, feta, and olives. Blend thoroughly. Place a lettuce leaf on each of four plates. Place one-fourth of the couscous salad in the center of each. Cut remaining three tomatoes into eight wedges each. Peel and slice cucumbers. Decoratively arrange tomato and cucumber slices around couscous. Squeeze lime juice over tomatoes and cucumber; sprinkle with pepper.

THREE-RICE SALAD WITH ALMONDS AND PEAS

Serves 4

Total calories per serving: 348
Total fat per serving: 5.9 g (15%)

3 cups water
1 6-ounce box Uncle Ben's Long
  Grain & Wild Rice with
  seasoning packet
½ cup long-grain white rice
2 tablespoons low-sodium soy
  sauce
1 tablespoon plus 2 teaspoons
  dark brown sugar
2 teaspoons cider vinegar
½ teaspoon grated fresh ginger
⅛ teaspoon black pepper
⅛ teaspoon cayenne pepper
½ 10-ounce package frozen peas,
  thawed
⅓ cup chopped onion
½ cup sliced water chestnuts
3 tablespoons chopped red bell
  pepper
⅓ cup sliced almonds, toasted in
  broiler
4 lettuce leaves

1. In a medium-sized saucepan, bring water to a boil. Add boxed rice, seasoning packet, and white rice. Return to a boil, stir, reduce heat, cover tightly, and simmer for 20 minutes. Remove from heat and let stand, covered, for 5 minutes. Cool completely.

2. In a small bowl, combine soy sauce, brown sugar, vinegar, ginger, black pepper, and cayenne.

3. At serving time, combine rice mixture, soy sauce mixture, peas, onion, water chestnuts, bell pepper, and almonds. Toss lightly but thoroughly. Place lettuce leaves on four plates, spoon equal amounts of rice salad on each, and serve immediately.

PEPPERED LIME SOUP, MOZZARELLA TORTILLA WEDGES, AND BLACK-EYED PEA SALAD

Serves 4

Total calories per serving: 338
Total fat per serving: 7.7 g (21%)

PEPPERED LIME SOUP *(81 calories, 1.2 g fat per serving)*

2 16-ounce cans chicken broth
1 cup chopped yellow onion
2½ tablespoons fresh lime juice
2 cloves garlic, minced
¼ teaspoon hot red pepper flakes
⅛ teaspoon chili powder
Dash black pepper
1 small tomato, seeded and
  chopped
⅓ cup cooked white rice, no
  butter, margarine, or oil used
  in cooking
2 teaspoons extra-virgin olive oil
⅛ teaspoon salt
4 teaspoons minced radish
4 teaspoons minced fresh cilantro
  leaves

1. In a 2-quart saucepan, bring broth to a boil. Add onion, lime juice, garlic, red pepper flakes, chili powder, and black pepper. Return to a boil, reduce heat, cover tightly, and simmer for 20 minutes. Stir in tomato, rice, oil, and salt. Remove from heat and let stand for 10 minutes. Flavors are enhanced if soup is refrigerated overnight.

2. At serving time, divide evenly among four soup bowls and top each with 1 teaspoon radish and 1 teaspoon cilantro. Serve immediately.

MOZZARELLA TORTILLA WEDGES *(139 calories, 5.6 g fat per serving)*

4 6-inch corn tortillas
1 cup (¼ pound) grated
  mozzarella cheese

1. Preheat oven to 475°F.
2. Sprinkle each tortilla with ¼ cup of the cheese, covering as much of the surface as possible. Place on two baking sheets and bake for 4 minutes or until cheese is melted and just beginning to brown. Remove from oven, cut each into six wedges, and serve immediately.

(Continued on the next page)

BLACK-EYED PEA SALAD *(118 calories, 0.9 g fat per serving)*

1 16-ounce can black-eyed peas,
  well rinsed and drained
1 cup chopped fresh tomato
½ cup chopped red onion
½ cup chopped cucumber,
  peeled if desired
¼ cup chopped celery
2 tablespoons chopped fresh
  parsley
2 tablespoons plus 2 teaspoons
  white wine vinegar
2 tablespoons plus 2 teaspoons
  semisweet white wine
1 teaspoon sugar
¼ teaspoon curry powder
¼ teaspoon chili powder
¼ teaspoon black pepper
¼ teaspoon salt
1 teaspoon Louisiana hot sauce
  or to taste

Combine all ingredients in a mixing bowl, toss well, cover, and refrigerate overnight or for at least 4 hours.

SPICED JAMAICAN CHILI WITH RICE

Serves 4

Total calories per serving: 345
Total fat per serving: 5.6 g (15%)

Cooking spray
½ pound lean ground round
2 cups chopped yellow onion
8 cloves garlic, minced
½ medium-sized green bell
  pepper, chopped
½ medium-sized red bell pepper,
  chopped
½ 16-ounce can dark red kidney
  beans, well rinsed and drained
2 16-ounce cans tomatoes,
  undrained, chopped
1 tablespoon chili powder
1 teaspoon ground cinnamon
½ teaspoon ground allspice
½ teaspoon ground cumin
⅛ teaspoon ground nutmeg
1 teaspoon beef bouillon granules
2 cups hot cooked rice, no salt or
  margarine used in cooking
¼ cup nonfat sour cream
¼ cup chopped scallions
Louisiana hot sauce to taste

1. Coat a large nonstick skillet with cooking spray and place over medium-high heat. Add beef and brown. Drain on paper towels and wipe out skillet with paper towels.

2. Coat skillet with more cooking spray, add onion and garlic, and cook until onion is transparent, about 4–6 minutes.

3. Add green and red peppers, beans, tomatoes and their liquid, chili powder, cinnamon, allspice, cumin, nutmeg, and bouillon granules. Stir, cover tightly, and simmer very gently for 15 minutes. Remove and let stand for 15 minutes to blend flavors. Serve over ½ cup rice, topped with 1 tablespoon sour cream, 1 tablespoon scallions, and hot sauce to taste.

DINNERS

Skewered Fresh Tuna with Lime, Gingered Rice and Fruit and Pepper Salsa

*Charred Fish with Chunky Red Pepper–Olive Oil Sauce and Baked
Potatoes with Sour Cream and Scallions*

*Baked Fish with Pasta and Mediterranean Salsa and Pan-Roasted
Pole Beans with Olive Oil*

*Snapper on a Bed of Spinach-Cheese Sauce, Basil-Baked Tomatoes,
and Gingered Rice*

Shrimp Linguine and Olives with Sautéed Zucchini

*Spicy Crumb-Topped Chicken, Sweet Corn,
and Pineapple-Lime Gelatin Salad*

Roasted Garlic Chicken with Parsleyed Rice and Lemon-Crusted Asparagus

*Chicken Noodle Parmesan and Fresh Pear Salad
with Creamy Orange Dressing*

*Chicken with Vegetables over Egg Noodles and
Pineapple-Mandarin Gelatin Salad*

*Chicken in Rich Cheese Sauce with New Potatoes and
Steamed Vegetables and Sliced Tomatoes*

*Lemon-Mustard Chicken with Angel Hair Pasta and Fresh Asparagus
with Summer-Ripe Tomatoes*

Cajun Chicken and Rice, Marinated Cucumbers, and Broccoli Flowerets

Sliced Turkey with Fresh Mushroom Gravy, Whipped Potatoes,
Peppered Peas, and Apricot Halves

Open-Faced Turkey Meatball Sandwiches and Crisp Cabbage
Vinaigrette Salad

Turkey Ham and Black-Eyed Pea Soup with Crisp-Topped Corn Muffins

Beef Patties, Sautéed Vegetables, and Blue Cheese, New Potatoes,
and Endive Salad with Creamy Herb Dressing

Stir-Fried Beef and Mushrooms with Oyster Sauce and Sweet-Sour Salad

Eight-Minute Roast, Fresh Asparagus,
Hearts of Palm, and Artichoke Salad, and Rice with Parsley

Old West Stew and Cilantro Tossed Salad with Santa Fe Dressing

Skewered BBQ Pork with Bacon and Pineapple

Savory Seared Pork with Seasoned Vegetables and
Baked Potatoes with Sour Cream

Hot Pork and Fruit Stir-Fry with Broccoli Spears

Stir-Fried Pork with Dipping Sauce, Raisin Rice with Peanuts,
and Steamed Baby Carrots

Overstuffed Potatoes, Baby Carrots with Sour Cream and
Horseradish Sauce, and Oven-Grilled Vegetables

Bean-Stuffed Peppers with Rice and Tossed Salad with Olives and Tortillas

Vegetable Fusilli with Tomato, Olive, and Feta Salad

Italian Rice and Beans and Creamy Dijon Salad with Artichokes

Southern Comfort Vegetable Dinner with Crisp-Topped Corn Muffins

Vegetable Pasta Casserole, Fresh Mushrooms with
Red Wine Vinaigrette, and Broccoli Flowerets

Bayou Country Vegetable Gumbo, Cajun Tossed Salad,
and Crisp-Topped Corn Muffins

SKEWERED FRESH TUNA WITH LIME, GINGERED RICE AND FRUIT AND PEPPER SALSA

Serves 4

Total calories per serving: 353
Total fat per serving: 4.9 g (12%)

SKEWERED FRESH TUNA WITH LIME *(159 calories, 4.5 g fat per serving)*

2 tablespoons low-sodium soy
  sauce
2 tablespoons fresh lime juice
2 cloves garlic, minced
¼ teaspoon black pepper
4 ¼-pound tuna steaks (about 1
  inch thick), cut into 1-inch
  pieces
½ medium-sized green bell
  pepper
½ medium-sized onion, cut into
  eighths and separated
8 cherry tomatoes
Cooking spray
Lime wedges for garnish

1. Preheat the broiler.
2. Combine soy sauce, lime juice, garlic, and pepper; whisk together until well blended. Add tuna to soy mixture, toss well to coat, and marinate for ½ hour, turning frequently.
3. Alternating vegetables and tuna, thread eight 12-inch skewers, reserving marinade. Coat a broiler rack with cooking spray. Place skewers on rack and place on broiler pan. Broil no less than 5 inches from heat source for 4 minutes. Baste with marinade, turn, baste, and broil for 3 minutes longer or until opaque in center. Serve immediately with lime wedges.

GINGERED RICE *(92 calories, 0.2 g fat per serving)*

⅔ cup long-grain white rice
1 teaspoon grated fresh ginger
1 teaspoon butter-flavored Molly
  McButter

Prepare rice according to package directions (do not use butter, margarine, or oil in cooking). Add ginger and butter flavoring. Stir thoroughly and serve.

(Continued on the next page)

FRUIT AND PEPPER SALSA *(102 calories, 0.2 g fat per serving)*

1 16-ounce can juice-packed
   pineapple chunks, well drained
2 medium-sized navel oranges,
   sectioned and chopped
¼ cup chopped scallion
¼ cup thinly sliced red bell
   pepper
2 tablespoons chopped fresh
   cilantro
1 fresh jalapeño pepper, chopped
   fine
4 lettuce leaves

Cut pineapple chunks in half and place in a mixing bowl with oranges, scallion, red bell pepper, cilantro, and jalapeño. Toss well and chill for 1 hour. At serving time, place equal amounts on lettuce leaves and serve.

CHARRED FISH WITH CHUNKY RED PEPPER–OLIVE OIL SAUCE AND BAKED POTATOES WITH SOUR CREAM AND SCALLIONS

Serves 4

Total calories per serving: 400
Total fat per serving: 8.2 g (18%)

CHARRED FISH WITH CHUNKY RED PEPPER–OLIVE OIL SAUCE
(258 calories, 8.2 g fat per serving)

Olive oil–flavored cooking spray
1 tablespoon extra-virgin olive oil
6 cloves garlic, minced
2 red bell peppers, cut into 1-inch pieces
1 green bell pepper, cut into 1-inch pieces
¾ cup chicken broth
2 tablespoons dry white wine
¼ teaspoon paprika
¼ teaspoon black pepper
¼ teaspoon salt
¼ cup water
2 6-ounce fillets grouper or any mild, lean white fish
1 tablespoon chili powder
1 tablespoon margarine (not light)
4 lemon wedges

1. *Be sure your kitchen is well ventilated before you prepare this dish.*
2. Coat a large nonstick skillet with cooking spray, add oil and garlic, and place over medium heat for 1 minute. Add peppers and cook for 10 minutes. Add broth, wine, paprika, and pepper. Cover tightly, reduce heat, and simmer until peppers are *very tender* and have a chunky sauce appearance, about 40–50 minutes, stirring occasionally. Stir in salt and water, stir to blend, cover, and set aside.
3. Rub both sides of fillets with chili powder. Place a cast-iron skillet over high heat until *very* hot.
4. Add margarine, melt, tilting pan to cover bottom, and add fillets. Cook for 2 minutes, turn, and cook for 2 minutes longer. Remove from heat and let stand *in skillet* for 3–4 minutes longer or until opaque in center.
5. If you wish, add 1–2 tablespoons water to peppers at this time, stirring to blend. Place fillets on individual plates, squeeze lemon juice over fish, spoon peppers and sauce around outer edges of fish, and serve immediately.

(Continued on the next page)

BAKED POTATOES WITH SOUR CREAM AND SCALLIONS
(142 calories, 0 g fat per serving)

4 6-ounce baking potatoes
½ cup nonfat sour cream
½ cup chopped scallions

1. Preheat oven to 350°F.
2. Bake potatoes for 50–60 minutes, or until easily pierced by a fork. Split lengthwise and gently push ends of each potato to open. Top each with 2 tablespoons sour cream and 2 tablespoons scallions and serve.

BAKED FISH WITH PASTA AND MEDITERRANEAN SALSA AND PAN-ROASTED POLE BEANS WITH OLIVE OIL

Serves 4

Total calories per serving: 399
Total fat per serving: 8.2 g (19%)

BAKED FISH WITH PASTA AND MEDITERRANEAN SALSA
(322 calories, 4.7 g fat per serving)

Salsa
4 medium-sized plum tomatoes, seeded and chopped
20 small black olives, pitted and sliced
2 teaspoons drained capers
3 tablespoons finely chopped yellow onion
1 tablespoon chopped fresh parsley
3 tablespoons red wine vinegar
½ teaspoon dried basil leaves
⅛ teaspoon salt
Dash of black pepper

Fish and Pasta
Cooking spray
1½ pounds fillets red snapper or any other mild, lean white fish
2 tablespoons fresh lemon or lime juice
Black pepper to taste
Paprika to taste
3 cups hot cooked linguine, no butter, margarine, or oil used in cooking
2 teaspoons light margarine
4 teaspoons freshly grated Parmesan cheese

1. In a small bowl, combine all salsa ingredients. Let stand for 30 minutes.
2. Preheat oven to 350°F.
3. Coat a 13″ × 9″ baking pan with cooking spray. Arrange fillets in a single layer in pan. Drizzle lemon juice over fish and sprinkle with black pepper and paprika. Cover and bake for 20–22 minutes or until opaque in center.
4. Place fillets on four plates, spoon salsa on top, and serve each with ¾ cup cooked pasta tossed with ½ teaspoon margarine and 1 teaspoon Parmesan.

(Continued on the next page)

PAN-ROASTED POLE BEANS WITH OLIVE OIL *(77 calories, 3.5 g fat per serving)*

1¼ pounds pole beans, trimmed and cut into 2-inch pieces
2 cloves garlic, minced
3 tablespoons minced yellow onion
½ teaspoon dried oregano leaves
2½ teaspoons extra-virgin olive oil
Black pepper to taste
Olive oil–flavored cooking spray
⅛ teaspoon salt

1. In a medium-sized mixing bowl, combine beans, garlic, onion, oregano, olive oil, and pepper. Toss well to blend thoroughly.
2. Coat a large nonstick skillet with cooking spray and place over medium-high heat for 1 minute. Add bean mixture and cook for 25–30 minutes or until tender, stirring occasionally. Sprinkle with salt, toss, and serve.

SNAPPER ON A BED OF SPINACH-CHEESE SAUCE, BASIL-BAKED TOMATOES, AND GINGERED RICE

Serves 4

Total calories per serving: 388
Total fat per serving: 7.1 g (16%)

SNAPPER ON A BED OF SPINACH-CHEESE SAUCE (247 calories, 6.2 g fat per serving)

4 6-ounce fillets red snapper
2 tablespoons fresh lemon juice
¼ teaspoon chili powder
Paprika to taste
¼ teaspoon black pepper
1 10-ounce package frozen
    chopped spinach
3 ounces Velveeta light cheese,
    cut into small pieces
2 teaspoons minced onion
2 cloves garlic, minced
½ teaspoon Worcestershire sauce
⅛ teaspoon cayenne pepper
⅛ teaspoon salt
¼ cup skim milk
1½ teaspoons cornstarch
Cooking spray
Lemon wedges for garnish

1. Preheat oven to 350°F.
2. Rinse fillets, pat dry with paper towels, and place in a 9″ × 13″ baking pan. Sprinkle lemon juice over fillets and top with chili powder, paprika, and ⅛ teaspoon black pepper. Cover tightly and set aside.
3. Cook spinach, without salt, according to package directions. Reserve ¼ cup of the cooking liquid, then drain spinach in a colander, squeezing out excess liquid by pressing down with paper towels.
4. Place spinach and reserved cooking liquid in a medium-sized saucepan. Add cheese, onion, garlic, Worcestershire, remaining ⅛ teaspoon black pepper, cayenne, and salt. In a small container, combine milk and cornstarch and blend until smooth. Add to spinach mixture and stir well. Place over medium-low heat and cook until cheese has melted completely.
5. Coat a 1-quart casserole dish with cooking spray, add spinach mixture, cover, and bake for 20 minutes, baking tomatoes at the same time. Add fish to oven with spinach and continue baking for 10 minutes. Remove spinach, uncover (spinach will have a soupy appearance at this point), and stir well. Let stand to thicken while fish continues to cook for 10 minutes longer or until opaque in center. Remove fish from oven. Spoon one-fourth of the spinach mixture onto each of four dinner plates. Using back of a spoon, spread sauce to cover a 6-inch diameter. Using a slotted spatula, place fish on top. Serve immediately with lemon wedges.

(Continued on the next page)

BASIL-BAKED TOMATOES *(49 calories, 0.7 g fat per serving)*

4 medium-sized tomatoes, halved
1 tablespoon plus 1 teaspoon
  fresh lemon juice
1 slice light bread, toasted and
  grated
1 tablespoon freshly grated
  Parmesan cheese
2 teaspoons minced fresh parsley
½ teaspoon dried basil leaves
Olive oil–flavored cooking spray

Crumple a sheet of foil and place on bottom of a baking sheet, to keep tomatoes balanced evenly, then set tomato halves on top. Spoon ½ teaspoon lemon juice on each tomato half. In a small bowl, combine bread crumbs, Parmesan, parsley, and basil. Toss to blend thoroughly. Sprinkle evenly over tomatoes and lightly spray cooking spray over all. Set aside while preparing snapper (see recipe on previous page), then bake along with fish for 20–25 minutes or until *just* tender.

GINGERED RICE *(92 calories, 0.2 g fat per serving)*

⅔ cup long-grain white rice
1 teaspoon grated fresh ginger
1 teaspoon butter-flavored Molly
  McButter

Prepare rice according to package directions (do not use butter, margarine, or oil in cooking). Add ginger and butter flavoring. Stir thoroughly and serve.

SHRIMP LINGUINE AND OLIVES WITH SAUTEED ZUCCHINI

Serves 4

Total calories per serving: 384
Total fat per serving: 10.8 g (25%)

SHRIMP LINGUINE AND OLIVES (353 calories, 9.5 g fat per serving)

Butter-flavored cooking spray
4 cloves garlic, minced
6 ounces mushrooms, sliced (about 2 cups)
½ cup chopped scallion
½ medium-sized red bell pepper, sliced thin
½ teaspoon dried Italian seasoning
¼ teaspoon black pepper
2 tablespoons dry red wine
3 medium-sized plum tomatoes, cut into 8 wedges each
10 ounces shrimp, peeled
16 small black olives, pitted and quartered
2 tablespoons chopped fresh parsley
1 tablespoon plus 1 teaspoon extra-virgin olive oil
¼ teaspoon salt
5 cups hot cooked linguine, no butter, margarine, or oil used in cooking
¼ cup freshly grated Parmesan cheese

1. Coat a large nonstick skillet with cooking spray. Place over medium-high heat for 1 minute. Add garlic and mushrooms and cook for 4 minutes or until mushrooms are beginning to brown.

2. Add scallion, bell pepper, Italian seasoning, and black pepper; cook for 3 minutes.

3. Add wine, tomatoes, and shrimp and cook for 5–6 minutes or until shrimp is done.

4. Add olives, parsley, oil, and salt and stir well. Add linguine and 2 tablespoons of the Parmesan; toss to blend. Place equal amounts on four dinner plates and top each with 1½ teaspoons Parmesan cheese. Serve immediately.

(Continued on the next page)

SAUTEED ZUCCHINI *(31 calories, 1.3 g fat per serving)*

1 pound zucchini, cut into
  julienne strips
¼ cup finely chopped onion
2 cloves garlic, minced
1 teaspoon extra-virgin olive oil
Butter-flavored cooking spray
¼ teaspoon salt

In a large mixing bowl, combine zucchini, onion, garlic, and oil. Toss well to coat thoroughly. Liberally coat a large nonstick skillet with cooking spray and place over medium-high heat for 1 minute. Add zucchini mixture and cook, stirring, for 7–8 minutes or until richly browned and tender. Sprinkle with salt and toss well. Serve immediately.

SPICY CRUMB-TOPPED CHICKEN, SWEET CORN, AND PINEAPPLE-LIME GELATIN SALAD

Serves 4

Total calories per serving: 400
Total fat per serving: 11.6 g (26%)

SPICY CRUMB-TOPPED CHICKEN *(200 calories, 7.8 g fat per serving)*

1 tablespoon plus 2 teaspoons light margarine at room temperature
2 teaspoons extra-virgin olive oil
2 teaspoons Worcestershire sauce
1 teaspoon fresh lemon juice
⅛ teaspoon garlic powder
½ teaspoon dry mustard
¼ teaspoon salt
⅛ teaspoon black pepper
1½ slices light bread, grated (not toasted)
Cooking spray
4 ¼-pound boneless chicken breast halves

1. Preheat the broiler.
2. In a small bowl, combine margarine, oil, Worcestershire sauce, lemon juice, garlic powder, dry mustard, salt, and pepper. Whisk until smooth. Using a fork, gently but thoroughly mix in soft bread crumbs.
3. Coat a broiler rack with cooking spray and place in broiler pan. Place chicken on rack and spoon one-fourth of the bread crumb mixture onto each chicken piece. Using a fork, spread mixture on top to coat evenly. Broil no less than 5 inches from heat source for 5½ minutes only. Remove from heat and let stand for 2 minutes to finish cooking. Serve immediately.

SWEET CORN *(98 calories, 0.1 g fat per serving)*

3 cups fresh or frozen white corn
4 teaspoons butter-flavored Molly McButter
Black pepper to taste

Lightly steam or boil corn until it is tender yet crisp. Transfer corn to a mixing bowl and stir in butter flavoring. Place ¾ cup corn on each of four plates, sprinkle with pepper, and serve.

(Continued on the next page)

PINEAPPLE-LIME GELATIN SALAD *(102 calories, 3.7 g fat per serving)*

1 3-ounce package sugar-free
  lime gelatin
⅔ cup boiling water
1 8-ounce can undrained juice-
  packed crushed pineapple
⅔ cup nonfat cottage cheese
¼ cup evaporated skim milk
⅓ cup fat-free mayonnaise-style
  salad dressing
1 tablespoon prepared
  horseradish
3 tablespoons (¾ ounce) pecan
  pieces, *lightly* browned in
  broiler

In a mixing bowl, combine lime gelatin and boiling water. Stir until gelatin dissolves. Add pineapple and its juices; stir well. Add cottage cheese, evaporated milk, salad dressing, and horseradish. Mix thoroughly, pour into a decorative bowl, and chill until set. At serving time, sprinkle pecans evenly over gelatin and serve.

ROASTED GARLIC CHICKEN WITH PARSLEYED RICE AND LEMON-CRUSTED ASPARAGUS

Serves 4

Total calories per serving: 400
Total fat per serving: 10 g (23%)

ROASTED GARLIC CHICKEN WITH PARSLEYED RICE (311 calories, 5.5 g fat per serving)

4 ½-pound chicken breast halves
8 cloves garlic, split in half lengthwise
4 teaspoons fresh lemon juice
¼ teaspoon salt
⅛ teaspoon black pepper
Paprika to taste
2 cups hot cooked rice, no butter, margarine, or salt used in cooking
2 teaspoons butter-flavored Molly McButter
3 tablespoons chopped fresh parsley

1. Preheat oven to 350°F.
2. Pull back skin from each chicken piece, place four garlic halves on meat, drizzle with 1 teaspoon lemon juice, and sprinkle with salt, pepper and paprika. Carefully rest skin on top and place on a wire rack in a baking pan. Bake for 45 minutes or until no longer pink in center and discard skin. Discard garlic if desired. Sprinkle lightly with more pepper.
3. Toss rice with butter flavoring and parsley. Place ¼ of the rice onto each of four serving plates. Top each with one chicken breast halve and serve.

LEMON CRUSTED ASPARAGUS (89 calories, 4.5 g fat per serving)

1 pound fresh asparagus
Butter-flavored cooking spray
3 tablespoons light margarine
1 tablespoon plus 1 teaspoon grated lemon zest
¼ teaspoon garlic powder
2 slices light bread, grated (not toasted)
¼ teaspoon salt
5 lemon wedges

1. Lightly steam asparagus until tender yet crisp. Keep warm.
2. Liberally coat a large nonstick skillet with cooking spray. Add margarine, lemon zest, and garlic powder and place over medium-high heat. Cook, stirring frequently, until it bubbles (about 2 minutes). Add bread crumbs and stir until golden, about 5–6 minutes. Add salt to bread crumbs.
3. Place warm asparagus in a decorative bowl, sprinkle with juice of 1 lemon wedge, top with bread crumb mixture, squeeze remaining lemon wedges over all, and serve immediately.

CHICKEN NOODLE PARMESAN AND FRESH PEAR SALAD WITH CREAMY ORANGE DRESSING

Serves 4

Total calories per serving: 400
Total fat per serving: 5.9 g (13%)

CHICKEN NOODLE PARMESAN *(294 calories, 5.4 g fat per serving)*

3½ cups water
2 16-ounce cans chicken broth
2 celery ribs, cut into 2-inch
   pieces
1 small onion, quartered
1 bay leaf
2 ½-pound skinless chicken breast
   halves
6 ounces extra-wide egg noodles
¼ cup skim milk
1 tablespoon cornstarch
⅛ teaspoon black pepper
3 tablespoons freshly grated
   Parmesan cheese
Freshly ground black pepper to
   taste

1. In a dutch oven, preferably cast iron, combine water, broth, celery, onion, and bay leaf. Bring to a boil, add chicken, return to a boil, reduce heat, cover tightly, and simmer for 25 minutes. Remove chicken, set aside to cool slightly, and remove bones. Discard celery, onion, and bay leaf. Defat broth.

2. Bring broth to a boil, add noodles, return to a boil, and cook, uncovered, for 10 minutes or until tender, stirring occasionally.

3. In a small container, combine milk and cornstarch and mix until cornstarch dissolves. Add black pepper and stir into noodles. Add chicken, reduce heat, and simmer until slightly thickened.

4. Remove from heat, sprinkle with Parmesan cheese, cover, and let stand for 10 minutes. Sprinkle with pepper and serve.

FRESH PEAR SALAD WITH CREAMY ORANGE DRESSING
(106 calories, 0.5 g fat per serving)

¼ cup frozen orange juice
   concentrate, thawed
3 tablespoons nonfat sour cream
1¼ teaspoons honey
4 lettuce leaves
2 pears, cored and sliced thin
1 cup seedless red or green grapes

1. In a small bowl, combine juice concentrate, sour cream, and honey. Whisk to blend thoroughly and chill until serving time.

2. Place a lettuce leaf on each of four salad plates. Decoratively arrange one-fourth the pear slices on top, spoon one-fourth of the dressing over pears, and top with grapes. Serve immediately.

CHICKEN WITH VEGETABLES OVER EGG NOODLES AND PINEAPPLE-MANDARIN GELATIN SALAD

Serves 4

Total calories per serving: 394
Total fat per serving: 4.6 g (11%)

CHICKEN WITH VEGETABLES OVER EGG NOODLES (306 calories, 4.5 g fat per serving)

1 16-ounce can chicken broth
1 cup chopped yellow onion
6 ounces mushrooms, quartered (about 2 cups)
½ cup thinly sliced celery
⅓ cup thinly sliced green bell pepper
1 bay leaf
¼ teaspoon paprika
Black pepper to taste
¾ pound skinless, boneless chicken breast, cut into 1-inch pieces
2 tablespoons cornstarch
½ teaspoon salt
3 cups hot cooked egg noodles, no butter, margarine, or oil used in cooking

1. In a large skillet, preferably cast iron, bring all but 2 tablespoons broth to a boil. Add onion, mushrooms, celery, bell pepper, bay leaf, paprika, pepper, and chicken. Return to a boil, stir, reduce heat, cover tightly, and simmer for 18 minutes. In a small container, combine cornstarch and remaining 2 tablespoons broth and stir until blended thoroughly. Stir into chicken mixture with salt and cook, uncovered, until thickened. Remove bay leaf.

2. Place ¾ cup noodles on each of four plates, spoon one-fourth of the chicken mixture on top of each, and sprinkle lightly with more pepper if desired.

(Continued on the next page)

PINEAPPLE-MANDARIN GELATIN SALAD *(88 calories, 0.1 g fat per serving)*

1 3-ounce package sugar-free
   orange gelatin
½ cup boiling water
5 ice cubes
1 8-ounce can juice-packed
   crushed pineapple, drained
   and juice reserved
1 cup vanilla nonfat yogurt
½ 11-ounce can mandarin
   oranges packed in light syrup,
   well drained

In a heatproof bowl, combine gelatin and boiling water and stir until gelatin dissolves. Add ice cubes and reserved pineapple juice. Stir until ice has completely melted. Place in freezer for 8 minutes or until it just begins to thicken. Remove and whisk in yogurt until well blended. Stir in pineapple and mandarin oranges. Spoon into four individual bowls, return to freezer, chill until set, about 10–12 minutes, and serve.

Variation: Place gelatin mixture in an 8-inch square glass pan and place in freezer for 40 minutes or until firm. Cut into fourths and place on lettuce to serve.

CHICKEN IN RICH CHEESE SAUCE WITH NEW POTATOES AND STEAMED VEGETABLES AND SLICED TOMATOES

Serves 4

Total calories per serving: 400
Total fat per serving: 7 g (16%)

¼ cup all-purpose flour
½ teaspoon ground cinnamon
⅛ teaspoon ground nutmeg
⅛ teaspoon black pepper
4 ¼-pound boneless chicken breast halves
Butter-flavored cooking spray
2 teaspoons light margarine
⅜ teaspoon salt
1 cup skim milk
1 tablespoon plus 1 teaspoon cornstarch
2½ ounces Velveeta light cheese, cut into small pieces (about ⅓ cup)
Dash cayenne pepper
8 2-ounce new potatoes, boiled until tender and halved
1½ cups cauliflower flowerets, steamed
1½ cups broccoli flowerets, steamed
Paprika for garnish
2 large tomatoes

1. Preheat oven to 325°F.
2. In a small bowl, combine flour, cinnamon, nutmeg, and pepper and mix thoroughly. Rinse and pat chicken dry; coat with flour mixture.
3. Liberally coat a large nonstick skillet with cooking spray, add margarine, and place over medium-high heat until bubbly. Stir to coat bottom of skillet. Add chicken, cook for 3 minutes, turn, and cook for 3 minutes longer. Transfer chicken to an 8″ × 12″ glass baking dish, sprinkle with ⅛ teaspoon salt, and bake for 10 minutes, uncovered.
4. While chicken is cooking, combine milk and cornstarch in a small bowl and stir until cornstarch dissolves. Pour into skillet over medium heat, stirring with a spatula, and cook until thickened. Add cheese, cayenne, and remaining ¼ teaspoon salt and stir until cheese melts. Remove from heat. Arrange potatoes, cauliflower, and broccoli around chicken and pour sauce over all. Sprinkle with paprika and bake, uncovered, for 5 minutes longer.
5. Thinly slice tomatoes. Remove chicken from oven and place equal amounts, along with one-fourth of the tomato slices, onto each of four plates. Serve.

LEMON-MUSTARD CHICKEN WITH ANGEL HAIR PASTA AND FRESH ASPARAGUS WITH SUMMER-RIPE TOMATOES

Serves 4

Total calories per serving: 395
Total fat per serving: 8.6 g (20%)

LEMON-MUSTARD CHICKEN WITH ANGEL HAIR PASTA
(300 calories, 6.6 g fat per serving)

2 tablespoons chopped scallion
1 tablespoon fresh lemon juice
2 tablespoons dry white wine
3 tablespoons chopped fresh
   parsley
2 teaspoons Dijon mustard
¼ cup chicken broth
Olive oil–flavored cooking spray
4 ¼-pound skinless, boneless
   chicken breast halves, flattened
   to ¼-inch thickness
2 teaspoons extra-virgin olive oil
1 tablespoon light margarine
¼ teaspoon salt
⅛ teaspoon black pepper
3 cups hot cooked angel hair
   pasta, no butter, margarine, or
   oil used in cooking

1. In a small bowl, combine scallion, lemon juice, wine, parsley, mustard, and broth. Mix well and set aside.
2. Coat a large nonstick skillet with cooking spray and place over high heat for 1 minute. Add chicken and cook for 2 minutes. Turn and cook for 2½ minutes longer. Set aside on a serving platter. Reduce heat to medium-high, add scallion mixture, and stir until smooth, scraping bottom and sides. Stir in oil, margarine, salt, and pepper. Blend well. Pour sauce over chicken, arrange pasta around chicken, and serve immediately.

FRESH ASPARAGUS WITH SUMMER-RIPE TOMATOES *(95 calories, 2 g fat per serving)*

4 cups chopped fresh asparagus
4 medium-sized ripe tomatoes
4 teaspoons light margarine

1. Lightly steam asparagus until tender yet crisp. While asparagus is cooking, thinly slice tomatoes. Decoratively place one-fourth of the slices onto each of four small plates. Set aside.
2. Mix together asparagus and margarine. Place 1½ cups asparagus on each plate. Serve.

CAJUN CHICKEN AND RICE, MARINATED CUCUMBERS, AND BROCCOLI FLOWERETS

Serves 4

Total calories per serving: 395
Total fat per serving: 5.8 g (13%)

CAJUN CHICKEN AND RICE *(308 calories, 4 g fat per serving)*

Cooking spray
4 6-ounce skinless chicken breast
　halves
4 cloves garlic, minced
⅔ cup long-grain white rice
1 cup chopped yellow onion
½ cup chopped green bell pepper
½ cup chopped scallion
½ cup chopped fresh parsley
½ teaspoon dried thyme leaves
2 tablespoons dry white wine
1 16-ounce can chicken broth
1 16-ounce can tomatoes,
　chopped and drained
2 teaspoons Worcestershire sauce
⅛ teaspoon cayenne pepper
¼ teaspoon salt
¼ teaspoon paprika
¼ teaspoon black pepper
Louisiana hot sauce to taste (if
　desired)

1. Preheat oven to 350°F.
2. Coat a dutch oven, preferably cast iron, with cooking spray and place over medium-high heat for 1 minute. Brown chicken pieces (meat side only) and set aside. Add garlic and rice to pan drippings and cook, stirring frequently with a spatula, for 5 minutes or until dark brown in color.
3. Add onion, bell pepper, scallion, parsley, thyme, wine, broth, tomatoes, Worcestershire sauce, and cayenne; stir well. Place chicken on top and gently press it down so it is surrounded by rice. Top with salt, paprika, and pepper. Cover tightly and bake for 45 minutes. Remove from oven and let stand for 15 minutes. At serving time, sprinkle with hot sauce if desired.

(Continued on the next page)

MARINATED CUCUMBERS *(38 calories, 0.3 g fat per serving)*

3 cups peeled and sliced
  cucumber
½ cup thinly sliced green or red
  bell pepper
½ cup thinly sliced red onion
¾ cup bottled fat-free Italian
  salad dressing
2 tablespoons Louisiana hot
  sauce or to taste
Black pepper to taste

In a decorative bowl, combine cucumber slices, bell pepper, and onion. In a small container, combine salad dressing, hot sauce, and pepper. Mix well and pour over cucumber mixture. Toss and refrigerate for 30 minutes before serving.

BROCCOLI FLOWERETS *(49 calories, 1.5 g fat per serving)*

3 cups fresh or frozen broccoli
  flowerets
4 teaspoons light margarine

1. Lightly steam broccoli until tender yet crisp. While broccoli is cooking, melt margarine.
2. Mix together broccoli and margarine and serve immediately.

SLICED TURKEY WITH FRESH MUSHROOM GRAVY, WHIPPED POTATOES, PEPPERED PEAS, AND APRICOT HALVES

Serves 4

Total calories per serving: 399
Total fat per serving: 6.1 g (14%)

SLICED TURKEY WITH FRESH MUSHROOM GRAVY *(157 calories, 3.5 g fat per serving)*

Butter-flavored cooking spray
2 cloves garlic, minced
2 cups (6 ounces) sliced
   mushrooms
¼ cup chopped scallion
2 tablespoons plus 2 teaspoons
   all-purpose flour
1 16-ounce can chicken broth
1 small bay leaf
Black pepper to taste
¾ pound roasted turkey breast
   meat, sliced and warmed

1. Coat a large nonstick skillet with cooking spray and place over medium-high heat for 1 minute. Add garlic and cook for 15 seconds. Add mushrooms and cook for 6–7 minutes or until edges begin to brown. Reduce heat to medium, stir in scallion, sprinkle flour evenly over mushrooms and scallion and toss well. Slowly stir in broth and continue stirring until well blended. Add bay leaf. Increase to medium-high heat, bring to a boil, and stir, using a spatula. Reduce heat and simmer for 10–12 minutes or until thickened, stirring frequently. Remove bay leaf and sprinkle with black pepper.

2. Place 3 ounces turkey on each of four plates. Spoon one-fourth of the gravy over turkey and potatoes.

WHIPPED POTATOES *(118 calories, 1.1 g fat per serving)*

1 quart water
1 pound white potatoes, peeled
   and cut into 1-inch pieces
½ cup skim milk
2 teaspoons light margarine
½ teaspoon butter-flavored Molly
   McButter
¼ teaspoon salt

1. Bring water to a boil in a saucepan, add potatoes, return to a boil, reduce heat, and simmer for 20 minutes.

2. Drain potatoes and place in a mixing bowl. Using an electric mixer on high speed, mash potatoes until smooth. Add milk, margarine, butter flavoring, and salt and blend thoroughly. Cover and keep warm.

(Continued on the next page)

PEPPERED PEAS *(64 calories, 1.5 g fat per serving)*

2 cups fresh or frozen young
  green peas
1 tablespoon light margarine
¼ teaspoon black pepper
¼ teaspoon sugar

1. Lightly steam peas until tender yet crisp.
2. While peas are cooking, melt margarine in a medium-sized saucepan over low heat. Add pepper and sugar and stir until sugar is dissolved. Reduce heat to very low.
3. Place warm peas in saucepan. Stir to coat peas with sauce.

APRICOT HALVES *(60 calories, 0 g fat per serving)*

2 cups juice-packed canned
  apricot halves

Serve ½ cup apricot halves with juice in each of four small bowls.

OPEN-FACED TURKEY MEATBALL SANDWICHES AND CRISP CABBAGE VINAIGRETTE SALAD

Serves 4

Total calories per serving: 388
Total fat per serving: 10.3 g (24%)

OPEN-FACED TURKEY MEATBALL SANDWICHES (356 calories, 7.9 g fat per serving)

⅔ pound lean ground turkey breast

1 10-ounce package frozen chopped spinach, thawed and squeezed dry

1 slice light bread, toasted and grated

¼ cup finely chopped yellow onion

2 tablespoons chopped fresh parsley

2 cloves garlic, minced

1 large egg white

½ teaspoon dried basil leaves

½ teaspoon dried oregano leaves

¼ teaspoon ground nutmeg

⅛ teaspoon ground allspice

¼ teaspoon black pepper

1 teaspoon beef bouillon granules

1 tablespoon hot water

Cooking spray

Paprika to taste

2 cups bottled low-fat spaghetti sauce

½ pound Italian bread, split lengthwise

½ cup (2 ounces) grated part-skim mozzarella cheese

2 tablespoons plus 2 teaspoons freshly grated Parmesan cheese

1. Preheat the broiler.

2. In a mixing bowl, combine turkey, spinach, bread crumbs, onion, parsley, garlic, egg white, basil, oregano, nutmeg, allspice, and pepper. In a small container, dissolve bouillon granules in hot water and add to turkey mixture. Mix well. Shape into 32 balls.

2. Coat broiler rack and pan with cooking spray. Place meatballs on rack and broil no less than 5 inches from heat source for 3 minutes. Turn, sprinkle with paprika, and broil for 4 minutes longer.

3. Place meatballs in a medium-sized nonstick skillet and pour spaghetti sauce over them. Bring to a boil, reduce heat, cover lightly, and simmer for 20 minutes.

4. Place a 2-ounce slice of bread on each plate, spoon eight meatballs with sauce on top of bread, and sprinkle each with 2 tablespoons mozzarella and 2 teaspoons Parmesan.

Variation: Prepare sandwiches on a baking sheet and broil for 1–2 minutes, no less than 5 inches from heat source, to melt mozzarella before serving. Then top with Parmesan.

(Continued on the next page)

CRISP CABBAGE VINAIGRETTE SALAD *(32 calories, 2.4 g fat per serving)*

2 teaspoons red wine vinegar
2 teaspoons extra-virgin olive oil
⅛ teaspoon garlic powder
⅛ teaspoon salt
⅛ teaspoon black pepper
2 cups shredded green cabbage
1 cup shredded red cabbage

1. In a small bowl, combine vinegar, oil, garlic powder, salt, and pepper. Whisk to blend thoroughly.
2. In a mixing bowl, combine green and red cabbage and dressing. Toss well to blend thoroughly. Serve immediately.

TURKEY HAM AND BLACK-EYED PEA SOUP WITH CRISP-TOPPED CORN MUFFINS

Serves 4

Total calories per serving: 398
Total fat per serving: 8.3 g (19%)

TURKEY HAM AND BLACK-EYED PEA SOUP *(294 calories, 4.8 g fat per serving)*

2 16-ounce cans chicken broth
1 cup chopped yellow onion
½ cup chopped green bell pepper
½ cup chopped carrot
3 cloves garlic, minced
½ teaspoon dried oregano leaves
½ teaspoon dry mustard
½ teaspoon chili powder
¼ teaspoon cayenne pepper
¼ teaspoon black pepper
1 16-ounce can black-eyed peas
2 medium-sized tomatoes
6 ounces turkey ham, sliced thin
   and chopped (about 1½ cups)
2 teaspoons Worcestershire sauce

1. In a dutch oven, preferably cast iron, bring broth to a boil. Add onion, bell pepper, carrot, garlic, oregano, dry mustard, chili powder, cayenne, and black pepper. Return to a boil, reduce heat, cover tightly, and simmer for 4 minutes.
2. Rinse and drain peas. Seed and coarsely chop tomatoes.
3. Add peas, tomatoes, turkey ham, and Worcestershire sauce, bring to a simmer, and cook for 4 minutes longer. Remove from heat and let stand for 20 minutes to blend flavors.

CRISP-TOPPED CORN MUFFINS *(104 calories, 3.5 g fat per serving)*

⅔ cup all-purpose flour
½ cup yellow cornmeal
2 teaspoons sugar
2 teaspoons baking powder
¼ teaspoon baking soda
¼ teaspoon salt
¾ cup plus 1 tablespoon nonfat
   buttermilk
1 large egg white
2 teaspoons vegetable oil
Cooking spray
4 teaspoons light margarine

1. Preheat oven to 450°F.
2. In a mixing bowl, combine flour, cornmeal, sugar, baking powder, baking soda, and salt. Whisk together until well blended. In a separate bowl, whisk together buttermilk, egg white, and oil. Place a nonstick muffin tin with at least eight cups in the oven and heat for 3 minutes.
3. Meanwhile, make a well in center of dry ingredients, pour buttermilk mixture into well, and stir until *just* blended. Remove muffin tin from oven, quickly coat with cooking spray, fill eight of the muffin cups, and bake for 15 minutes. Immediately remove muffins from pan and serve each with 1 teaspoon margarine. Remaining muffins may be stored in an airtight container for up to one week.

BEEF PATTIES, SAUTEED VEGETABLES, AND BLUE CHEESE, NEW POTATOES, AND ENDIVE SALAD WITH CREAMY HERB DRESSING ·

Serves 4

Total calories per serving: 384
Total fat per serving: 9.6 g (23%)

BEEF PATTIES, SAUTEED VEGETABLES, AND BLUE CHEESE
(234 calories, 9.2 g fat per serving)

1 pound lean ground round
2 cloves garlic, minced
Cooking spray
1 tablespoon plus 1 tcaspoon
    Worcestershire sauce
Paprika to taste
½ pound mushrooms, sliced
1 medium-sized green bell
    pepper, sliced thin
1 medium-sized yellow onion,
    sliced thin
¼ cup water
2 tablespoons dry red wine
¼ teaspoon salt
¼ teaspoon black pepper
2 tablespoons (1 ounce)
    crumbled blue cheese

1. Preheat the broiler.
2. Combine beef and garlic and shape into four patties. Coat a broiler rack and pan with cooking spray and set patties on rack. Broil 2–3 inches from heat source for 3 minutes. Turn, spoon ½ teaspoon Worcestershire sauce over each patty, sprinkle each with paprika, and broil for 3 minutes longer. Place on a serving platter.
3. Coat a large skillet, preferably cast iron, with cooking spray and place over medium-high heat for 1 minute. Add mushrooms and cook for 4 minutes. Add bell pepper and onion and cook for 6–7 minutes longer or until edges *just* begin to brown. Combine water, wine, salt, pepper, and remaining 2 teaspoons Worcestershire sauce and pour over vegetables in skillet. Stir well and cook for 1 minute longer.
4. Spoon equal amounts of vegetables and any liquid over beef patties and top with crumbled cheese. Serve immediately.

NEW POTATOES *(109 calories, 0 g fat per serving)*

8 new potatoes (about 12 ounces)
4 tablespoons nonfat sour cream
4 tablespoons chopped scallion

1. Preheat oven to 350°F.
2. Bake potatoes for 25–35 minutes or until easily pierced with a fork. Place two potatoes on each of four small plates, top each serving with 1 tablespoon sour cream and 1 tablespoon scallions, and serve.

ENDIVE SALAD WITH CREAMY HERB DRESSING *(41 calories, 0.4 g fat per serving)*

Dressing

1 cup nonfat buttermilk
¼ cup fat-free mayonnaise-style salad dressing
¼ cup nonfat sour cream
1 tablespoon grated onion
1 tablespoon minced fresh parsley
1 teaspoon fresh lemon juice
½ teaspoon dry mustard
½ teaspoon black pepper
½ teaspoon dried thyme leaves
¼ teaspoon salt
¼ teaspoon garlic powder

Salad

2 cups torn endive leaves
2 cups mixed salad greens such as red leaf, Boston, and Bib lettuce
2 medium-sized tomatoes, cut into eighths
¼ cup sliced red onion
½ cup sliced cucumber, peeled if desired
Freshly ground black pepper to taste

1. Combine all dressing ingredients in a small bowl and whisk until smooth. Chill.

2. In a salad bowl, combine endive, mixed greens, tomatoes, onion, and cucumber. Add ½ cup of the salad dressing, toss gently but thoroughly to coat, and serve immediately with freshly ground black pepper. Remaining dressing may be refrigerated for up to two weeks, but not past the expiration date of the buttermilk, mayonnaise, and sour cream.

STIR-FRIED BEEF AND MUSHROOMS WITH OYSTER SAUCE AND SWEET-SOUR SALAD

Serves 4

Total calories per serving: 398
Total fat per serving: 11.1 g (25%)

STIR-FRIED BEEF AND MUSHROOMS WITH OYSTER SAUCE
(329 calories, 8.1 g fat per serving)

½ cup canned condensed beef broth
¼ cup bottled oyster sauce
1 tablespoon cornstarch
1 teaspoon sugar
2 tablespoons dry sherry
2 tablespoons water
2 tablespoons low-sodium soy sauce
Cooking spray
1 tablespoon vegetable oil
2 cloves garlic, minced
1 teaspoon grated fresh ginger
¾ pound lean top round, cut into very thin strips
½ pound mushrooms, quartered (about 3 cups)
½ cup thinly sliced yellow onion
½ cup thinly sliced green bell pepper
½ 8-ounce can bamboo shoots, well drained
3 cups hot cooked rice, no butter, margarine, or oil used in cooking

1. In a small bowl, combine broth, oyster sauce, cornstarch, sugar, sherry, water, and soy sauce. Blend well and set aside.

2. Coat a large nonstick skillet with cooking spray, add 1 teaspoon of the oil, and place over high heat. Add garlic and ginger and cook for 15 seconds. Add half of the beef and stir-fry for 2–3 minutes. Remove with a slotted spoon and set aside. Add remaining beef, cook for 2–3 minutes, and set aside.

3. Heat remaining 2 teaspoons oil in skillet. Add mushrooms, onion, and bell pepper and cook for 4 minutes. Add bamboo shoots, reserved beef, and broth mixture. Stir well and cook until thickened, about 2 minutes. Immediately serve each portion over ¾ cup rice.

SWEET-SOUR SALAD *(69 calories, 3 g fat per serving)*

Dressing

¼ cup white wine vinegar

2 tablespoons plus 2 teaspoons dark brown sugar

2 tablespoons low-sodium soy sauce

2 teaspoons vegetable oil

1 teaspoon dry mustard

½ teaspoon ground ginger

¼ teaspoon garlic powder

¼ teaspoon hot red pepper flakes

Salad

4 cups fresh spinach leaves

½ cup thinly sliced red bell pepper

½ cup chopped scallion

½ 8-ounce can sliced water chestnuts, well drained and slivered

1 tablespoon plus 1 teaspoon sesame seeds, toasted

1. In a small bowl, combine all dressing ingredients and whisk until well blended. Chill. (Dressing may be refrigerated for up to two months.)

2. In a salad bowl, decoratively arrange spinach, bell pepper, scallion, and water chestnuts. Chill.

3. At serving time, add ⅓ cup of the dressing to salad. Toss gently yet thoroughly to coat. Top with toasted sesame seeds and serve immediately.

EIGHT-MINUTE ROAST, FRESH ASPARAGUS, HEARTS OF PALM, AND ARTICHOKE SALAD, AND RICE WITH PARSLEY

Serves 4

Total calories per serving: 390
Total fat per serving: 9 g (21%)

EIGHT-MINUTE ROAST *(183 calories, 5 g fat per serving)*

1¼ pounds lean eye of round
   roast, trimmed of all fat
½ cup lite teriyaki sauce
½ teaspoon barbecue smoke
   seasoning
Cooking spray

1. Place roast in a small narrow bowl. Combine teriyaki sauce and smoke seasoning. Mix well, pour over roast, and marinate overnight in refrigerator.
2. Preheat oven to 500°F. Coat a baking pan with cooking spray and place roast on a wire rack in pan, discarding marinade. Bake for 8 minutes only, turn off oven, and leave beef in oven for 6 hours. Do not open oven door. At serving time, slice thin.

FRESH ASPARAGUS, HEARTS OF PALM, AND ARTICHOKE SALAD
(117 calories, 4 g fat per serving)

1½ cups fresh asparagus, cut into
   2-inch pieces and steamed
   lightly
½ 16-ounce can hearts of palm,
   well drained and cut into 1-
   inch pieces
½ 14-ounce can artichoke hearts,
   well drained and quartered
4 plum tomatoes, each cut
   crosswise into 8 slices
4 thin slices red onion, separated
   into rings
3 tablespoons cider vinegar
1 tablespoon vegetable oil
1 tablespoon semisweet white
   wine
2 teaspoons sugar
1 clove garlic, minced
½ teaspoon black pepper

1. Place asparagus, hearts of palm, artichoke hearts, tomatoes, and onion in a decorative bowl.
2. Combine vinegar, oil, wine, sugar, garlic, and pepper. Whisk together until well blended. Pour over vegetables and toss gently but thoroughly to coat. Refrigerate (for up to 6 hours) until serving time.

RICE WITH PARSLEY *(90 calories, 0 g fat per serving)*

2 cups hot cooked rice, no
    butter, margarine, or oil used
    in cooking
1 tablespoon chopped fresh
    parsley

Toss rice and parsley together and serve.

OLD WEST STEW AND CILANTRO TOSSED SALAD WITH SANTE FE DRESSING

Serves 4

Total calories per serving: 400
Total fat per serving: 10.2 g (23%)

OLD WEST STEW *(367 calories, 9.9 g fat per serving)*

Butter-flavored cooking spray
1 pound lean boneless chuck roast, trimmed of all fat and cut into 1-inch pieces
2 tablespoons all-purpose flour
2½ cups plus 2 tablespoons water
1 medium-sized yellow onion, cut into eighths
1 10-ounce can condensed beef broth
¼ cup dry red wine
2 cloves garlic, minced
½ teaspoon dried thyme leaves
1 bay leaf
½ teaspoon salt
¼ teaspoon black pepper
1 pound white potatoes, peeled and cut into 1-inch pieces
4 medium-sized carrots, cut into 2-inch pieces
1 celery rib, cut into 1-inch pieces
½ cup thinly sliced green bell pepper
1 tablespoon Worcestershire sauce
2 tablespoons cornstarch
2 tablespoons chopped fresh parsley

1. Coat a dutch oven, preferably cast iron, with cooking spray and place over high heat for 1 minute. Add beef and brown on all sides, stirring constantly until juices are released. Sprinkle flour evenly over meat and stir to coat thoroughly. Add 2½ cups of the water, onion, beef broth, wine, garlic, thyme, bay leaf, salt, and pepper. Bring to a boil, reduce heat, cover tightly, and simmer for 1 hour and 15 minutes.

2. Increase heat to high and add potatoes, carrots, celery, bell pepper, and Worcestershire. Bring to a boil, stir, reduce heat, cover tightly, and simmer for 20 minutes, stirring occasionally.

3. In a small container, combine cornstarch with remaining 2 tablespoons water, mixing until cornstarch dissolves. Add to pot along with parsley, stir well, and cook, uncovered, for 10 minutes longer. Remove bay leaf and serve.

CILANTRO TOSSED SALAD WITH SANTE FE DRESSING *(33 calories, 0.3 g fat per serving)*

Dressing
¾ cup medium Pace picante
   sauce
⅓ cup nonfat sour cream
1 tablespoon plus 1 teaspoon
   fresh lime juice
1½ teaspoons sugar
½ teaspoon chili powder

Salad
4 cups mixed salad greens
½ cup sliced cucumber, peeled if
   desired
½ cup thinly sliced green bell
   pepper
½ cup thinly sliced celery
¼ cup chopped red onion
2 tablespoons chopped fresh
   cilantro leaves
2 small radishes, sliced thin
Freshly ground black pepper to
   taste

1. Combine all dressing ingredients in a small bowl and whisk to mix thoroughly. Chill.

2. In a salad bowl, decoratively arrange salad greens, cucumber, bell pepper, celery, onion, cilantro, and radishes. Chill until serving time.

3. At serving time, add ½ cup salad dressing and toss gently yet thoroughly to coat. Place salad on individual plates and sprinkle with black pepper. Remaining dressing may be refrigerated for up to two weeks, but not past the expiration date of the sour cream.

SKEWERED BBQ PORK WITH BACON AND PINEAPPLE

Serves 4

Total calories per serving: 388
Total fat per serving: 6.6 g (15%)

¾ pound pork tenderloin, cut into 1-inch pieces

¼ cup low-sodium soy sauce

⅓ cup bottled barbecue sauce

½ 8-ounce can juice-packed crushed pineapple, undrained

4 slices lower-sodium bacon, each cut into 8 pieces

1 medium-sized green bell pepper, cut into 1-inch pieces

1 medium-sized yellow onion, cut into 8 wedges and separated

1 8-ounce can juice-packed pineapple slices, well drained and cut into bite-sized pieces

Cooking spray

3 cups hot cooked rice, no butter, margarine, or oil used in cooking

1. In a shallow bowl, combine pork and soy sauce. Toss well, cover, and refrigerate overnight or for at least 2 hours, turning occasionally.

2. Preheat the broiler.

3. In a food processor, combine barbecue sauce and crushed pineapple and process until smooth.

4. Drain pork and discard marinade. On eight 12-inch skewers, alternate pork, bacon, bell pepper, onion, and pineapple. Coat a broiler rack and pan with cooking spray, place rack in pan, and arrange skewers on top. Spoon half of the barbecue mixture evenly over all and broil 2–3 inches away from heat source for 3 minutes. Turn skewers, spoon remaining sauce over all, and broil for 3 minutes longer or until bacon is done. Immediately serve each person two skewers and ¾ cup rice.

SAVORY SEARED PORK WITH SEASONED VEGETABLES AND BAKED POTATOES WITH SOUR CREAM

Serves 4

Total calories per serving: 370
Total fat per serving: 11.7 g (28%)

SAVORY SEARED PORK *(180 calories, 8.7 g fat per serving)*

Butter-flavored cooking spray
8 2-ounce boneless lean thin center-cut pork loin cutlets, trimmed of all fat
Garlic powder to taste
Salt to taste
Cayenne pepper to taste
Black pepper to taste

1. Preheat oven to warm.
2. Coat a large nonstick skillet with cooking spray and place over medium-high heat for 1 minute. Add four of the cutlets and sprinkle with garlic powder, salt, cayenne pepper, and black pepper. Cook for 1½ minutes, turn, and sprinkle with seasonings again, if desired. Cook for 1½–2 minutes longer. Place on a platter and set in oven. Repeat with remaining cutlets and serve immediately.

SEASONED VEGETABLES *(48 calories, 3 g fat per serving)*

2 tablespoons light margarine, softened
¼ teaspoon chili powder
1½ teaspoons Louisiana hot sauce
¼ teaspoon garlic powder
½ teaspoon fresh lime or lemon juice
2 cups broccoli flowerets, steamed
1 cup carrots, cut into julienne strips and steamed
1 cup cauliflower flowerets, steamed

In a small bowl, combine margarine, chili powder, hot sauce, garlic powder, and lime juice. Using an electric mixer, beat until well blended. Chill thoroughly. At serving time, spread chilled butter mixture over hot vegetables, allowing it to melt.

BAKED POTATOES WITH SOUR CREAM *(142 calories, 0 g fat per serving)*

4 6-ounce baking potatoes
½ cup nonfat sour cream

1. Preheat oven to 350°F.
2. Bake potatoes for 50–60 minutes until easily pierced by a fork. Split lengthwise. Push ends to open. Top with 2 tablespoons sour cream. Serve.

HOT PORK AND FRUIT STIR-FRY WITH BROCCOLI SPEARS

Serves 4

Total calories per serving: 372
Total fat per serving: 8.1 g (20%)

HOT PORK AND FRUIT STIR-FRY *(334 calories, 8.1 g fat per serving)*

Cooking spray
1 pound pork tenderloin, cut into
   thin strips
2 cloves garlic, minced
½ teaspoon grated fresh ginger
¼–½ teaspoon hot red pepper
   flakes, to taste
1 tablespoon vegetable oil
2 medium-sized yellow onions,
   cut into eighths and separated
½ cup thinly sliced red bell
   pepper
12 dried apricots, sliced thin
6 dried prunes, sliced thin
½ cup drained sliced water
   chestnuts, slivered
2 tablespoons low-sodium soy
   sauce
2 tablespoons water
1 teaspoon sugar
⅛ teaspoon black pepper
2 cups hot cooked rice, no
   butter, margarine, or oil used
   in cooking

1. Coat a large nonstick skillet with cooking spray and place over high heat for 1 minute. Add pork, garlic, ginger, and red pepper flakes. Cook, stirring constantly, until browned and no longer pink in center; set aside.

2. Reduce heat to medium-high, add oil and onions, and cook, stirring, for 3 minutes. Add red bell pepper and stir. Add apricots, prunes, and water chestnuts and stir. Add soy sauce, water, sugar, and black pepper; stir and cook for 30 seconds. Place ½ cup rice on each plate and top with equal amounts of pork mixture.

BROCCOLI SPEARS *(38 calories, 0 g fat per serving)*

1 pound fresh or frozen broccoli
   spears
1 tablespoon plus 1 teaspoon
   low-sodium soy sauce

Lightly steam broccoli until tender crisp. Place one-fourth of the broccoli on each of four plates. Sprinkle 1 teaspoon soy sauce over each serving of broccoli and serve.

STIR FRIED PORK WITH DIPPING SAUCE, RAISIN RICE WITH PEANUTS, AND STEAMED BABY CARROTS

Serves 4

Total calories per serving: 398
Total fat per serving: 7.3 g (17%)

¾ cup unsweetened pineapple juice
½ cup water
2 tablespoons plus 1½ teaspoons dry sherry
2 tablespoons plus 1½ teaspoons hoisin sauce
1½ teaspoons sugar
¾ teaspoon chili powder
3 tablespoons raisins, halved
3 tablespoons peanuts, toasted in broiler
3 tablespoons chopped scallion
2 tablespoons chopped red bell pepper
3 cups hot cooked rice, no butter, margarine, or oil used in cooking
2 cups baby carrots
Butter-flavored cooking spray
1 pound pork tenderloin, cut into thin strips
1 clove garlic, minced
⅛ teaspoon black pepper

1. In a small saucepan, combine pineapple juice, water, sherry, hoisin sauce, sugar, and chili powder. Bring to a boil, reduce heat, and simmer, uncovered, for 8 minutes. Set aside.

2. In a small bowl, combine raisins, peanuts, scallion, and bell pepper. Set aside.

3. Pour equal amounts of the dipping sauce into four small bowls. Combine raisin mixture and rice in a decorative bowl and toss to blend thoroughly. Cover to keep warm.

4. Lightly steam carrots until tender yet crisp. Keep warm.

5. Coat a large nonstick skillet with cooking spray and place over high heat for 1 minute. Add pork, garlic, and black pepper and stir-fry for 5 minutes or until all liquid is absorbed. Place one-fourth of the rice onto each of four plates. Top each with one-fourth of the pork. Place ½ cup carrots alongside rice and serve immediately.

OVERSTUFFED POTATOES, BABY CARROTS WITH SOUR CREAM AND HORSERADISH SAUCE, AND OVEN-GRILLED VEGETABLES

Serves 4

Total calories per serving: 396
Total fat per serving: 6.9 g (16%)

OVERSTUFFED POTATOES *(248 calories, 4.1 g fat per serving)*

4 ½-pound white potatoes, wrapped in foil
1 cup skim milk
½ cup evaporated skim milk
1 tablespoon light margarine
1 tablespoon butter-flavored Molly McButter
¾ teaspoon salt
⅛ teaspoon black pepper
⅛ teaspoon cayenne pepper
2 tablespoons finely chopped scallion
½ cup (2 ounces) grated reduced-fat sharp cheddar cheese
Paprika for garnish

1. Preheat oven to 350°F.
2. Bake potatoes for 1 hour and 15 minutes; leave oven on. Split lengthwise and scoop out potato, being careful not to tear skin. Place cooked potato in a mixing bowl. Using an electric mixer, beat potato until smooth. Add skim milk, evaporated milk, margarine, butter flavoring, salt, black pepper, and cayenne and beat until smooth. Beat in scallion.
3. Pile all of the potato mixture into potato skins, top each with 2 tablespoons grated cheese, sprinkle with paprika, and place on a foil-lined baking sheet. Bake for 5–8 minutes longer or until cheese melts.

BABY CARROTS WITH SOUR CREAM AND HORSERADISH SAUCE
(93 calories, 0.2 g fat per serving)

⅔ cup nonfat sour cream
3 tablespoons prepared horseradish
2 tablespoons plus 1 teaspoon skim milk
¼ teaspoon salt
⅛ teaspoon black pepper
1 pound baby carrots, steamed

Combine all ingredients except carrots in a small bowl and mix well. Chill thoroughly. At serving time, serve each person one-fourth of the carrots and spoon one-fourth of the sauce into four small individual bowls for dipping.

OVEN-GRILLED VEGETABLES *(55 calories, 2.6 g fat per serving)*

1 small zucchini, cut into ½-inch pieces
1 medium-sized yellow squash, cut into ½-inch pieces
½ medium-sized red bell pepper, cut into 1-inch pieces
1 medium-sized yellow onion, cut into 8 wedges
4 cloves garlic, minced
½ teaspoon dried Italian seasoning
1 tablespoon fresh lemon juice
2 teaspoons extra-virgin olive oil
⅛ teaspoon black pepper
Butter-flavored cooking spray
⅛ teaspoon salt

1. Preheat the broiler.
2. In a large mixing bowl, combine zucchini, yellow squash, bell pepper, and onion. In a small container, combine garlic, Italian seasoning, lemon juice, oil, and pepper. Whisk until well blended. Pour over vegetables and toss gently yet thoroughly to coat.
3. Liberally coat a broiler pan with cooking spray, place vegetables in pan in a single layer, and broil 2–3 inches from heat source for 6–7 minutes or until tender, stirring occasionally. Sprinkle with salt and serve.

BEAN–STUFFED PEPPERS WITH RICE AND TOSSED SALAD WITH OLIVES AND TORTILLAS

Serves 4

Total calories per serving: 397
Total fat per serving: 8.7 g (20%)

BEAN–STUFFED PEPPERS WITH RICE (278 calories, 2.9 g fat per serving)

1 cup well rinsed and drained canned pinto beans, ¼ cup liquid reserved
¼ cup chopped onion
1½ teaspoons chili powder
¼ teaspoon ground cumin
¼ teaspoon dried oregano leaves
2 cloves garlic, minced
½ teaspoon salt
⅛ teaspoon black pepper
⅛ teaspoon cayenne pepper
6 drops Louisiana hot sauce or to taste
3 tablespoons fresh lime juice
Cooking spray
1 cup long-grain white rice
¼ cup chopped fresh parsley
2 cups water
2 medium-sized green or red bell peppers, halved lengthwise and seeded
½ cup (2 ounces) grated reduced-fat sharp cheddar cheese
¼ cup chopped scallion
½ cup nonfat sour cream
½ cup seeded and chopped tomato

1. Preheat oven to 350°F.
2. In a food processor, combine beans, reserved liquid, onion, chili powder, cumin, oregano, garlic, salt, black pepper, cayenne, hot sauce, and 1 tablespoon of the lime juice. Blend until smooth.
3. Coat a 9-inch square baking dish with cooking spray. Add rice, parsley, water, and remaining 2 tablespoons lime juice and stir to blend thoroughly.
4. Arrange pepper halves in dish with rice and fill peppers with bean mixture. Cover tightly and bake for 45 minutes or until rice is cooked. Place 1 pepper half on each plate, surround it with one-fourth of the rice mixture, and top each pepper with 2 tablespoons cheese, 1 tablespoon scallion, 2 tablespoons sour cream, and 2 tablespoons tomato. Serve immediately.

TOSSED SALAD WITH OLIVES AND TORTILLAS *(119 calories, 5.8 g fat per serving)*

4 cups torn romaine and iceberg
  lettuce leaves
2 medium-sized tomatoes,
  chopped
½ cup Santa Fe Dressing (see
  Index)
24 small black olives, pitted and
  sliced thin
1½ ounces tortilla chips,
  crumbled (about 1 cup)

Place 1 cup torn lettuce leaves on each of four salad plates. Add one-fourth of the tomatoes, 2 tablespoons dressing, one-fourth of the olives, and one-fourth of the chips. Serve immediately.

VEGETABLE FUSILLI WITH TOMATO, OLIVE, AND FETA SALAD

Serves 4

Total calories per serving: 396
Total fat per serving: 12.9 g (29%)

VEGETABLE FUSILLI *(298 calories, 8.3 g fat per serving)*

Butter-flavored cooking spray
4 cloves garlic, minced
2 medium-sized zucchini, sliced thin
¾ pound mushrooms, quartered (about 4 cups)
1 cup chopped yellow onion
1 cup chopped red bell pepper
1 teaspoon dried basil leaves
1 teaspoon dried oregano leaves
⅜ teaspoon salt
⅛ teaspoon black pepper
4 cups hot cooked fusilli, no butter, margarine, or oil used in cooking
2 tablespoons chopped fresh parsley
1 tablespoon plus 1 teaspoon extra-virgin olive oil
2 tablespoons freshly grated Parmesan cheese

1. Coat a large nonstick skillet with cooking spray and place over medium-high heat for 1 minute. Add garlic, zucchini, mushrooms, onion, bell pepper, basil, and oregano. Cook for 10–12 minutes or until all liquid is evaporated and vegetables are just beginning to brown.

2. Add salt, pepper, pasta, and parsley and toss to blend thoroughly. Drizzle oil over all and toss again. Place equal amounts on four dinner plates and top each with 1½ teaspoons Parmesan cheese. Serve immediately.

TOMATO, OLIVE, AND FETA SALAD *(98 calories, 4.6 g fat per serving)*

4 lettuce leaves
8 ¾-inch-thick slices tomato
  (about 4 large)
4 teaspoons red wine vinegar or
  balsamic vinegar
¼ cup (2 ounces) crumbled feta
  cheese
1 tablespoon plus 1 teaspoon
  minced fresh parsley
16 small black olives, pitted and
  quartered
Freshly ground black pepper to
  taste

1. Place a lettuce leaf on each of four salad plates and top each with two tomato slices, overlapping slightly. Spoon ½ teaspoon vinegar over each slice, using back of a spoon to spread it evenly.

2. In a small bowl, combine cheese, parsley, and olives; toss well to blend thoroughly. Spoon equal amounts over tomato slices, top with pepper, and serve.

ITALIAN RICE AND BEANS AND CREAMY DIJON SALAD WITH ARTICHOKES

Serves 4

Total calories per serving: 389
Total fat per serving: 10.7 g (25%)

ITALIAN RICE AND BEANS (324 calories, 7.2 g fat per serving)

Olive oil–flavored cooking spray
1 tablespoon plus 2 teaspoons
   extra-virgin olive oil
¾ cup long-grain white rice
4 cloves garlic, minced
1½ cups chopped yellow onion
1 cup chopped fresh parsley
½ medium-sized green bell
   pepper, chopped
½ cup chopped scallion
1 teaspoon dried basil leaves
1 teaspoon dried oregano leaves
1 16-ounce can chicken broth
1 16-ounce can tomatoes, well
   drained, chopped
⅛ teaspoon black pepper
½ 16-ounce can navy beans, well
   rinsed and drained
½ teaspoon salt
2 tablespoons fresh lemon juice

1. Coat a dutch oven, preferably cast iron, with cooking spray, add 2 teaspoons of the oil, and place over medium-high heat for 1 minute. Add rice and garlic and cook for 7 minutes or until rice has turned a rich brown, stirring *constantly* to prevent scorching. Set aside in a bowl.

2. To dutch oven, add onion, ½ cup parsley, bell pepper, scallion, basil, and oregano. Cook, stirring frequently, for 4 minutes. Stir in broth, tomatoes, black pepper, and reserved rice. Reduce heat, cover, and simmer for 20 minutes. Stir in beans, salt, lemon juice, remaining 1 tablespoon oil, and remaining ½ cup parsley. Remove from heat, cover, and let stand for 10 minutes to allow flavors to blend.

CREAMY DIJON SALAD WITH ARTICHOKES *(65 calories, 3.5 g fat per serving)*

Dressing:
½ cup plain nonfat yogurt
1 tablespoon extra-virgin olive oil
1 tablespoon plus 1 teaspoon
   Dijon mustard
1 clove garlic, minced
½ teaspoon salt
¼ teaspoon pepper
1 tablespoon plus 1 teaspoon
   freshly grated Parmesan cheese

Salad
4 cups torn romaine lettuce
   leaves
¼ cup sliced red onion rings
4 water-packed canned artichoke
   hearts, quartered

1. Combine all dressing ingredients in a blender and blend until smooth. Chill.

2. Place 1 cup lettuce on each of four salad plates. Top with ¼ of the onion rings and four artichoke quarters. Drizzle 2 tablespoons dressing over each serving. Remaining dressing may be refrigerated for up to two weeks, but not past the expiration date of the yogurt.

SOUTHERN COMFORT VEGETABLE DINNER WITH CRISP-TOPPED CORN MUFFINS

Serves 4

Total calories per serving: 400
Total fat per serving: 5 g (11%)

YEAR-ROUND TURNIPS *(17 calories, 0 g fat per serving)*

1½ cups water
1 Knorr ham bouillon cube
1 16-ounce bag frozen chopped turnips
¼ teaspoon sugar
Louisiana hot sauce (if desired)

In a medium-sized saucepan, bring water to a boil. Add bouillon cube and mash and stir to dissolve. Add turnips and sugar. Return to a boil, stir, reduce heat, cover tightly, and simmer for 35 minutes. Remove from heat and let stand for 10 minutes to blend flavors. Serve with hot sauce if desired.

SLOW-SIMMERED BLACK-EYED PEAS *(119 calories, 0.8 g fat per serving)*

1 16-ounce can chicken broth
1 10-ounce package (about 2 cups) frozen black-eyed peas
½ ounce turkey ham, chopped fine (about ¼ cup)

In a medium-sized saucepan, bring broth to a boil, add black-eyed peas, return to a boil, reduce heat, cover tightly, and simmer for 50 minutes. Add ham and cook for 10 minutes longer or until beans are tender.

BAKED SWEET POTATOES *(102 calories, 0.4 g fat per serving)*

2 ½-pound sweet potatoes
2 teaspoons light margarine

1. Preheat oven to 350°F.
2. Bake potatoes for 1 hour and 10 minutes. Split in half lengthwise and serve each half with ½ teaspoon margarine.

CREAMY COUNTRY COLESLAW *(58 calories, 0.3 g fat per serving)*

4 cups shredded green cabbage
½ cup chopped onion
2 tablespoons sugar
½ teaspoon salt
⅛ teaspoon black pepper
¼ cup fat-free mayonnaise-style
    salad dressing
2 tablespoons cider vinegar

Place cabbage and onion in a mixing bowl and set aside. In a separate small bowl, combine sugar, salt, pepper, salad dressing, and vinegar; whisk together to blend thoroughly. Add to cabbage and stir well to coat thoroughly. Refrigerate for at least 1 hour before serving.

CRISP-TOPPED CORN MUFFINS *(104 calories, 3.5 g fat per serving)*

⅔ cup all-purpose flour
½ cup yellow cornmeal
2 teaspoons sugar
2 teaspoons baking powder
¼ teaspoon baking soda
¼ teaspoon salt
¾ cup plus 1 tablespoon nonfat
    buttermilk
1 large egg white
2 teaspoons vegetable oil
Cooking spray
4 teaspoons light margarine

1. Preheat oven to 450°F.
2. In a mixing bowl, combine flour, cornmeal, sugar, baking powder, baking soda, and salt. Whisk together until well blended. In a separate bowl, whisk together buttermilk, egg white, and oil. Place a nonstick muffin tin with at least eight cups in the oven and heat for 3 minutes.
3. Meanwhile, make a well in center of dry ingredients, pour buttermilk mixture into well, and stir until *just* blended. Remove muffin tin from oven, quickly coat with cooking spray, fill eight of the muffin cups, and bake for 15 minutes. Immediately remove muffins from pan and serve each with 1 teaspoon margarine. Remaining muffins may be stored in an airtight container for up to one week.

VEGETABLE PASTA CASSEROLE, FRESH MUSHROOMS WITH RED WINE VINAIGRETTE, AND BROCCOLI FLOWERETS

Serves 4

Total calories per serving: 400
Total fat per serving: 8.1 g (18%)

VEGETABLE PASTA CASSEROLE *(305 calories, 4.6 g fat per serving)*

Olive oil–flavored cooking spray
6 cloves garlic, minced
1 medium-sized green bell
   pepper, chopped
½ cup chopped yellow onion
1 16-ounce can tomatoes,
   undrained, chopped
½ cup water
⅓ cup chopped fresh parsley
1½ teaspoons dried basil leaves
1½ teaspoons dried oregano leaves
¼ teaspoon sugar
¼ teaspoon salt
⅛ teaspoon black pepper
Dash cayenne pepper
½ pound uncooked penne pasta
   noodles
½ cup (2 ounces) grated part-
   skim mozzarella cheese
2 tablespoons freshly grated
   Parmesan cheese

1. Preheat oven to 350°F.
2. Coat a dutch oven, preferably cast iron, with cooking spray and place over medium-high heat for 1 minute. Add garlic, bell pepper, and onion and cook for 7 minutes or until onion is transparent. Add tomatoes and their liquid, water, parsley, basil, oregano, sugar, salt, black pepper, cayenne, and pasta. Stir and blend well.
3. Cover tightly and bake for 35 minutes or until pasta is tender. Top with mozzarella and Parmesan cheeses and bake for 5 minutes longer. Remove from oven, uncover, and let stand for 5 minutes to blend flavors.

FRESH MUSHROOMS WITH RED WINE VINAIGRETTE *(46 calories, 2 g fat per serving)*

Dressing
¼ cup red wine vinegar
1 tablespoon extra-virgin olive oil
2 tablespoons dry white wine
2 tablespoons water
½ teaspoon dry mustard
½ teaspoon salt
¼ teaspoon black pepper
1 clove garlic, minced

Salad
3 cups torn red leaf lettuce
¼ cup chopped red onion
1 cup (3 ounces) sliced
  mushrooms
4 cherry tomatoes, halved
Freshly ground black pepper to
  taste

1. Combine all dressing ingredients in a blender and process until well blended. Chill.

2. In a salad bowl, combine lettuce, onion, and mushrooms. Pour ⅓ cup dressing over salad and toss gently yet thoroughly. Remaining dressing may be refrigerated for up to two weeks. Place equal amounts of salad on each of four salad plates with two tomato halves. Sprinkle with pepper and serve immediately.

BROCCOLI FLOWERETS *(49 calories, 1.5 g fat per serving)*

3 cups fresh or frozen broccoli
  flowerets
4 teaspoons light margarine

1. Lightly steam broccoli until tender yet crisp. While broccoli is cooking, melt margarine.

2. Mix together broccoli and margarine and serve immediately.

BAYOU COUNTRY VEGETABLE GUMBO, CAJUN TOSSED SALAD, AND CRISP-TOPPED CORN MUFFINS

Serves 4

Total calories per serving: 381
Total fat per serving: 5.4 g (13%)

BAYOU COUNTRY VEGETABLE GUMBO *(251 calories, 0.8 g fat per serving)*

¼ cup all-purpose flour
Butter-flavored cooking spray
2 cloves garlic, minced
2 cups chopped yellow onion
1 medium-sized green bell
  pepper, chopped
2 16-ounce cans chicken broth
10 fresh okra pods, cut into ½-
  inch pieces (about 1 cup)
½ cup chopped celery
1 16-ounce can tomatoes,
  undrained, chopped
2 bay leaves
¼ teaspoon dried oregano leaves
½ teaspoon dried thyme leaves
¼ teaspoon black pepper
⅛ teaspoon cayenne pepper
½ teaspoon Worcestershire sauce
Louisiana hot sauce to taste
¼ teaspoon sugar
¼ teaspoon salt
3 cups hot cooked rice, no
  butter, margarine, or oil used
  in cooking

1. Place a dutch oven, preferably cast iron, over medium-high heat, add flour, and brown, stirring constantly to prevent scorching, for 10 minutes. Immediately place flour on a sheet of foil and set aside.

2. Liberally coat dutch oven with cooking spray and add garlic, onion, and bell pepper. Cook for 5 minutes, stirring frequently. Sprinkle browned flour evenly over vegetables and toss to coat thoroughly. Slowly stir in broth.

3. Add okra, celery, tomatoes and their liquid, bay leaves, oregano, thyme, black pepper, cayenne, Worcestershire, hot sauce, sugar, and salt. Bring to a boil, stir well, reduce heat, cover tightly, and simmer for 2 hours, stirring occasionally with a spatula.

4. Remove from heat and let stand for 30 minutes to blend flavors and thicken slightly. Flavor improves if gumbo is allowed to refrigerate overnight. Serve each serving over ¾ cup rice.

CAJUN TOSSED SALAD *(26 calories, 1.1 g fat per serving)*

3½ cups torn mixed salad greens
½ cup shredded red cabbage
¼ cup chopped scallion
1 tablespoon chopped fresh
   parsley
½ cup bottled fat-free Italian
   salad dressing
1 tablespoon plus 1 teaspoon
   Louisiana hot sauce or to taste
¼ teaspoon sugar

In a salad bowl, combine greens, cabbage, scallion, and parsley. Set aside. In a small container, combine salad dressing, hot sauce, and sugar. Mix thoroughly and pour over salad. Toss gently but thoroughly to coat. Serve immediately.

CRISP-TOPPED CORN MUFFINS *(104 calories, 3.5 g fat per serving)*

⅔ cup all-purpose flour
½ cup yellow cornmeal
2 teaspoons sugar
2 teaspoons baking powder
¼ teaspoon baking soda
¼ teaspoon salt
¾ cup plus 1 tablespoon nonfat
   buttermilk
1 large egg white
2 teaspoons vegetable oil
Cooking spray
4 teaspoons light margarine

1. Preheat oven to 450°F.
2. In a mixing bowl, combine flour, cornmeal, sugar, baking powder, baking soda, and salt. Whisk together until well blended. In a separate bowl, whisk together buttermilk, egg white, and oil. Place a nonstick muffin tin with at least eight cups in the oven and heat for 3 minutes.
3. Meanwhile, make a well in center of dry ingredients, pour buttermilk mixture into well, and stir until *just* blended. Remove muffin tin from oven, quickly coat with cooking spray, fill eight of the muffin cups, and bake for 15 minutes. Immediately remove muffins from pan and serve each with 1 teaspoon margarine. Remaining muffins may be stored in an airtight container for up to one week.

DESSERTS

Fresh Lemon Sponge Cake with Glaze

Orange Spice Cupcakes with Pineapple Topping

Chocolate Mint Cupcakes

Raspberry-Kissed Pears in Phyllo Nests

Ladyfinger Strawberry Spokes

Fresh Melon and Grapes with Sweet Lime Cream

Phyllo Peach Packets

Tropical Cream Phyllo Tarts

Lemony Fresh Fruit Cookie Tarts

Sweet Blueberry–Filled Crepes Topped with Yogurt

Fresh Peaches with Strawberry Cream Cheese Dip

Banana-Ginger-Topped Frozen Yogurt

Lemon-Cream Fruit Parfaits

Springtime Strawberry Simplicity

Frozen Chocolate Mint Crumble

Peaches and Cream, Sherbet Style

Cinnamon-Steamed Apples with Caramel Sauce

Spiced Cranberry-Poached Pears

Chocolate-Crumbled Banana Crescents

Sparkling Ginger Fruit

Fruit Smoothies

Frozen Triple Cookies

Creamy Strawberry Orange Frost

Chocolate Freezer

Colossal Strawberry-Orange-Ginger Cooler

Tropical Snow Slush

Mixed Fruit Ice Pops

Spiced Apple and Citrus Warmer

Hot "Buttered" Grog

FRESH LEMON SPONGE CAKE WITH GLAZE

Serves 4

Total calories per serving: 99
Total fat per serving: 1.4 g (13%)

Cake
1 large egg yolk
2 tablespoons granulated sugar
2 teaspoons vanilla extract
1 tablespoon grated lemon zest
3 large egg whites at room
    temperature
¼ cup cake flour
½ teaspoon baking powder
⅛ teaspoon salt
Cooking spray

Glaze
2 tablespoons powdered sugar
1 teaspoon fresh lemon juice
½ teaspoon skim milk

1. Preheat oven to 350°F.
2. In a mixing bowl, combine egg yolk, granulated sugar, vanilla, and 1 tablespoon lemon zest; whisk until well blended.
3. In a separate bowl, using an electric mixer on high speed, beat egg whites until stiff peaks form. Gently but thoroughly fold into egg yolk mixture. A tablespoon at a time, fold in flour with baking powder and salt.
4. Coat an 8-inch square nonstick baking pan with cooking spray. Spoon batter evenly into pan and bake for 12 minutes. Place on a wire rack to cool completely.
5. In a small container, combine powdered sugar, lemon juice, and milk and whisk until smooth. When cake has cooled, top with glaze and serve.

ORANGE SPICE CUPCAKES WITH PINEAPPLE TOPPING

Makes 24

Total calories per serving: 100
Total fat per serving: 2.0 g (18%)

Cake
1 18-ounce box Duncan Hines
   Moist Deluxe Spice Cake Mix
1⅓ cups water
½ cup egg substitute
Juice of ½ medium-sized orange
   (2 tablespoons)
1 tablespoon grated orange zest
½ teaspoon vanilla butter nut
   flavoring
Cooking spray

Topping
¾ cup juice-packed crushed
   pineapple, undrained
1½ tablespoons water
1 teaspoon cornstarch

1. Preheat oven to 325°F.
2. In a mixing bowl, combine cake mix, 1⅓ cups water, egg substitute, orange juice, orange zest, and flavoring. Using an electric mixer, beat at low speed to blend, about 1 minute. Increase speed to medium and beat for 2 minutes longer, occasionally scraping sides and bottom with a rubber spatula.
3. Coat nonstick muffin tins with a total of 24 cups with cooking spray. Spoon batter evenly into cups. Bake for 17–18 minutes or until a wooden pick inserted in center of one cupcake comes out clean. Remove from oven and let cool on a rack for 5 minutes before removing from tins.
4. Meanwhile, prepare topping. In a medium-sized saucepan, combine pineapple, its juices, 1½ tablespoons water, and cornstarch. Stir until cornstarch dissolves. Place over medium-high heat and bring to a boil, stirring frequently. Boil for 15 seconds or until topping is beginning to thicken. Remove from heat and allow to cool.
5. When cake and pineapple have cooled, spoon approximately 1½ teaspoons of the pineapple mixture onto each cupcake. One cupcake equals one serving. Remaining cupcakes may be refrigerated in an airtight container for up to one week.

CHOCOLATE MINT CUPCAKES

Makes 24

Total calories per serving: 100
Total fat per serving: 1.7 g (15%)

1 18-ounce box Duncan Hines
    Moist Deluxe Chocolate
    Devil's Food Cake Mix
1⅓ cups cold water
½ cup egg substitute
1 teaspoon peppermint extract
2 tablespoons hot water
2 teaspoons instant coffee
    granules
Cooking spray

1. Preheat oven to 325°F.
2. In a mixing bowl, combine cake mix, cold water, egg substitute, and peppermint extract. In a small container, combine hot water and coffee granules; dissolve and add to batter.
3. Using an electric mixer, beat at low speed to blend, about 1 minute. Increase speed to medium and beat for 2 minutes longer, occasionally scraping sides and bottom with a rubber spatula.
4. Coat muffin tins with a total of 24 cups with cooking spray. Spoon batter evenly into cups. Bake for 16–18 minutes or until a wooden pick inserted in center of one cupcake comes out clean. Remove from oven and let cool on a wire rack for 5 minutes before removing from tins. One cupcake equals one serving. Remaining cupcakes may be stored in an airtight container for up to one week.

RASPBERRY-KISSED PEARS IN PHYLLO NESTS

Serves 4

Total calories per serving: 99
Total fat per serving: 0.5 g (5%)

1 sheet thawed frozen phyllo dough
Butter-flavored cooking spray
2 pears, peeled, cored, and halved lengthwise
2 tablespoons plus 2 teaspoons raspberry all-fruit spread
⅛ teaspoon almond extract
½ teaspoon powdered sugar

1. Preheat oven to 350°F.
2. Spray both sides of phyllo sheet with cooking spray. Working quickly, cut dough into four lengthwise strips and then cut each strip into fourths crosswise to make 16 squares. Coat a nonstick muffin tin with the cooking spray and place four squares in each of four tins, corners overlapping in center. Press down gently so dough takes the shape of the tin. Ruffle edges to create a nest appearance. Bake for 4 minutes. Remove from oven and cool completely in pan before removing gently and setting aside.
3. Place pears in a steamer basket over boiling water in a dutch oven. Cover tightly and steam for 6–8 minutes or until *just* tender. Remove from dutch oven and let cool slightly. Cut into ½-inch pieces and place equal amounts in phyllo nests.
4. Thirty minutes before serving, melt fruit spread over low heat, remove from heat, stir in almond extract, and quickly spoon 2 teaspoons melted spread over pear filling in each phyllo nest. Let stand for 20 minutes. Dust edges with powdered sugar and serve immediately.

LADYFINGER STRAWBERRY SPOKES

Serves 4

Total calories per serving: 99
Total fat per serving: 2.1 g (19%)

6 whole ladyfingers, split
3 tablespoons plus 2 teaspoons
   strawberry all-fruit spread,
   melted
¼ cup lite whipped topping
1 cup sliced strawberries

Arrange three ladyfinger halves on each of four dessert plates, forming a spoke design. Spoon ½ teaspoon melted strawberry spread onto each ladyfinger half, top each with 1 teaspoon whipped topping, and spread evenly over ladyfinger. Decoratively arrange ¼ cup strawberry slices on top of ladyfingers and drizzle 1¼ teaspoons melted strawberry spread over berries. Serve immediately or refrigerate until serving time.

FRESH MELON AND GRAPES WITH SWEET LIME CREAM

Serves 4

Total calories per serving: 100
Total fat per serving: 0.7 g (6%)

1 cup vanilla nonfat yogurt
2 tablespoons fresh lime juice
½ teaspoon grated lime zest
2 cups watermelon cubes
1 cup seedless green grapes
1 cup seedless red grapes
1½ cups honeydew cubes

1. Combine yogurt, lime juice, and zest. Whisk together until well blended and chill.
2. Decoratively arrange on each of four individual dessert plates ½ cup watermelon, ¼ cup green grapes, ¼ cup red grapes, and one-fourth of the honeydew. At serving time, spoon ¼ cup lime cream over each. Serve immediately.

PHYLLO PEACH PACKETS

Serves 4

Total calories per serving: 97
Total fat per serving: 0.3 g (3%)

1⅓ cups sliced peaches
1 tablespoon plus 1 teaspoon
  granulated sugar
½ teaspoon vanilla extract
½ teaspoon fresh lemon juice
¼ teaspoon ground cinnamon
2 sheets thawed frozen phyllo
  dough
Butter-flavored cooking spray
4 teaspoons peach all-fruit spread
1 teaspoon powdered sugar

1. Preheat oven to 375°F.
2. In a mixing bowl, combine peaches, granulated sugar, vanilla, lemon juice, and cinnamon. Toss gently yet thoroughly to coat.
3. Working with one phyllo sheet at a time (keep other sheet wrapped), lightly spray both sides with cooking spray. Cut in half, working quickly, and fold one half sheet in half crosswise. Place ⅓ cup of peach mixture in center and fold in edges, overlapping them to close up each packet. Place on a nonstick baking sheet and repeat process with second half of phyllo, working quickly to prevent dough from drying out. Repeat with other sheet.
4. Bake for 18 minutes. Remove from oven and let stand on a baking sheet for 5 minutes before removing. Carefully remove packets and place on individual dessert plates.
5. Melt peach spread over low heat (do not boil). Drizzle 1 teaspoon over each packet. Dust each with ¼ teaspoon powdered sugar and serve.

TROPICAL CREAM PHYLLO TARTS

Serves 4

Total calories per serving: 99
Total fat per serving: 1.3 g (12%)

1 sheet thawed frozen phyllo
dough

Butter-flavored cooking spray

¼ **3-ounce package sugar-free
vanilla pudding**

½ **cup skim milk**

7 **tablespoons lite whipped
topping**

2–3 **drops coconut extract (if
desired)**

¼ **cup juice-packed crushed
pineapple**

1 **medium-sized kiwi, peeled,
sliced, and halved**

½ **cup well-drained mandarin
oranges packed in light syrup**

4 **strawberries with stems**

½ **teaspoon powdered sugar**

1. Preheat oven to 350°F.

2. Spray both sides of phyllo sheet with cooking spray. Working quickly, cut dough into four lengthwise strips and then cut each strip into fourths crosswise to make 16 squares. Coat a nonstick muffin tin with the cooking spray and place four squares in each of four tins, corners overlapping in center. Press down gently so dough takes the shape of the tin. Ruffle edges to create a nest appearance. Bake for 4 minutes. Remove from oven and cool completely in pan before removing gently and setting aside.

3. In a small bowl, combine pudding mix with milk. Whisk together until smooth. Add whipped topping and coconut extract; fold together gently but thoroughly. Cover and chill until serving time.

4. At serving time, spoon one-fourth of the pudding mixture into each phyllo nest. Spoon 1 tablespoon of the crushed pineapple into center of each. Decoratively arrange one-fourth of the kiwi slices and 2 tablespoons of the mandarin oranges around outer edge of pineapple. Top each with one strawberry. Sprinkle edges of phyllo nest with powdered sugar and serve immediately.

LEMONY FRESH FRUIT COOKIE TARTS

Serves 4

Total calories per serving: 100
Total fat per serving: 2.6 g (23%)

¼ cup all-purpose flour
2½ teaspoons granulated sugar
2½ teaspoons margarine (*not light*)
1 teaspoon grated lemon zest
1 teaspoon fresh lemon juice
¼ teaspoon vanilla extract
Cooking spray
¼ cup nonfat vanilla yogurt
½ cup seedless green grapes, halved
½ medium-sized fresh nectarine, sliced thin
½ cup finely chopped fresh pineapple
½ medium-sized kiwi, halved and cut into 4 slices
¼ cup thinly sliced bananas
1 teaspoon powdered sugar

1. Preheat oven to 425°F.
2. In a food processor, combine flour, granulated sugar, margarine, lemon zest, lemon juice, and vanilla. Process until well blended. Roll dough into four balls, wrap with plastic wrap, and chill for 15 minutes. Removing one at a time from refrigerator, place a ball on a floured sheet of plastic wrap, cover with another sheet, and roll it into a 4-inch circle. Repeat process with remaining dough, coat two baking sheets with cooking spray, and place dough circles on baking sheets. Cover with foil and bake for 9–11 minutes or until edges just begin to brown. Cool completely on wire racks.
3. At serving time, spread 1 tablespoon yogurt evenly over each crust. Decoratively arrange on each cookie crust 2 tablespoons grapes, one-fourth of the nectarine, 2 tablespoons chopped pineapple, two pieces kiwi, and 1 tablespoon sliced banana. Dust each with ¼ teaspoon powdered sugar and serve immediately. (The crust is delicate and will dissolve if not served immediately after tarts are assembled.)

SWEET BLUEBERRY–FILLED CREPES TOPPED WITH YOGURT

Serves 4

Total calories per serving: 99
Total fat per serving: 0.4 g (4%)

Blueberry Filling
3 tablespoons frozen grape juice
    concentrate, thawed
2 teaspoons cornstarch
1 cup frozen blueberries, thawed
1 teaspoon vanilla extract

Crepes
⅓ cup plus 2 tablespoons skim
    milk
¼ cup all-purpose flour
1 teaspoon sugar
1 teaspoon vanilla extract
½ teaspoon grated lemon zest (if
    desired)
1 large egg white at room
    temperature
Butter-flavored cooking spray
¼ cup nonfat vanilla yogurt

1. In a small saucepan, combine grape juice concentrate and cornstarch. Whisk together until cornstarch dissolves. Place over medium-high heat, bring to a boil, and boil for 15 seconds, stirring frequently.

2. Remove from heat, pour over berries, add vanilla, and toss gently. Set aside for 10 minutes to blend flavors.

3. In a mixing bowl, combine milk, flour, sugar, vanilla, and lemon zest if desired. Whisk until smooth.

4. In a separate bowl, beat egg white, using an electric mixer on high speed, until stiff peaks form. Gently but thoroughly fold into milk mixture; batter will be slightly lumpy. Chill for at least 1 hour.

5. Coat a large nonstick skillet with cooking spray and place over medium heat for 1 minute. Gently stir mixture to blend thoroughly, then spoon ¼ cup batter into skillet and quickly tilt to spread batter evenly over skillet. Cook for 2 minutes, turn, and cook for 1½ minutes longer or until crepe no longer sticks on bottom. Place on a kitchen towel and repeat for the next three crepes. Fill each with one-fourth of the blueberry filling, fold edges over, and top each with 1 tablespoon yogurt.

FRESH PEACHES WITH STRAWBERRY CREAM CHEESE DIP

Serves 4

Total calories per serving: 99
Total fat per serving: 1 g (9%)

½ cup fat-free cream cheese
2 tablespoons plus 2 teaspoons
  strawberry all-fruit spread
2 tablespoons plus 2 teaspoons
  skim milk
½ cup lite whipped topping
3 medium-sized peaches,
  unpeeled, sliced thin
8 whole strawberries with stems

1. In a mixing bowl, combine cream cheese, strawberry spread, and milk. Using an electric mixer, blend until smooth. Gently but thoroughly fold in whipped topping. Chill until serving time.
2. Place one-fourth of the sweetened cream in center of each of four individual dessert plates. Decoratively arrange one-fourth of the peach slices around sweetened cream. Remove stems from four of the strawberries and cut into quarters. Evenly space four strawberry quarters around cream. Leaving stem ends attached, cut remaining strawberries to make fans and top each serving with a strawberry fan. Serve.

BANANA-GINGER-TOPPED FROZEN YOGURT

Serves 4

Total calories per serving: 97
Total fat per serving: 0.8 g (7%)

1 cup vanilla nonfat frozen
  yogurt
4 gingersnaps, crumbled
¾ cup thinly sliced bananas
Ground nutmeg or cinnamon for
  garnish

In each of four chilled wineglasses, place ¼ cup frozen yogurt. Top with one-fourth of the cookie crumbs and ¼ cup banana slices. Sprinkle lightly with nutmeg or cinnamon and serve immediately.

LEMON-CREAM FRUIT PARFAITS

Serves 4

Total calories per serving: 100
Total fat per serving: 1.3 g (12%)

1 3-ounce package sugar-free
    lemon gelatin
1 cup boiling water
8 ice cubes
¼ cup nonfat buttermilk
2 tablespoons fat-free cream
    cheese
1 teaspoon vanilla extract
2 teaspoons fresh lemon juice
½ teaspoon grated lemon zest
2 tablespoons powdered sugar
½ cup lite whipped topping
¼ cup juice-packed crushed
    pineapple, well-drained
1 cup thinly sliced bananas
1 cup quartered strawberries

1. In a mixing bowl, combine gelatin and boiling water. Stir until gelatin dissolves completely. Add ice cubes and stir until melted. Pour equal amounts into four parfait glasses or wineglasses. Chill until set.
2. In a mixing bowl, combine buttermilk, cream cheese, vanilla, lemon juice, lemon zest, and powdered sugar. Using an electric mixer, blend until smooth. Spoon equal amounts over set gelatin. Top each with 2 tablespoons whipped topping, 1 tablespoon crushed pineapple, ¼ cup banana slices, and ¼ cup strawberries and serve.

SPRINGTIME STRAWBERRY SIMPLICITY

Serves 4

Total calories per serving: 99
Total fat per serving: 0.3 g (3%)

1⅓ cups vanilla nonfat frozen
  yogurt
2 cups sliced strawberries
2 teaspoons powdered sugar
4 strawberries with stems

In each of four dessert bowls, place ⅓ cup frozen yogurt. Top each with ½ cup sliced strawberries, dust with ½ teaspoon powdered sugar, and top with a whole strawberry. Serve immediately.

FROZEN CHOCOLATE MINT CRUMBLE

Serves 4

Total calories per serving: 98
Total fat per serving: 1.4 g (13%)

1 chocolate graham cracker,
  crushed
2 peppermint candies, crushed
1⅓ cups chocolate nonfat frozen
  yogurt
6 tablespoons lite whipped
  topping

1. Combine graham cracker crumbs and crushed peppermints in a small bowl and toss to mix thoroughly.
2. Place ⅓ cup frozen yogurt in each of four dessert cups, sprinkle half of the crumb mixture evenly over all, top each with 1½ tablespoons whipped topping, and top all with remaining half of crumb mixture. Serve immediately or place in freezer until serving time.

PEACHES AND CREAM, SHERBET STYLE

Serves 4

Total calories per serving: 98
Total fat per serving: 0.2 g (2%)

1 16-ounce bag frozen
    unsweetened sliced peaches
3 tablespoons plus 2 teaspoons
    apricot all-fruit spread
½ cup vanilla nonfat yogurt

In a food processor, combine all ingredients and blend until smooth. Spoon into dessert dishes and serve immediately for a creamier texture or place in freezer for 45 minutes for a lightly frozen sherbet texture. Stir gently and serve immediately.

CINNAMON-STEAMED APPLES WITH CARAMEL SAUCE

Serves 4

Total calories per serving: 95
Total fat per serving: 0.6 g (6%)

4 medium-sized Red Delicious
    apples
3 cups water
Apple pie spice or ground
    cinnamon to taste
1 tablespoon plus 1 teaspoon
    bottled caramel ice cream
    topping

1. Using a vegetable peeler, peel apples. Cut apples in half and core. Place cut side down in a steamer basket. Add water to a dutch oven, place steamer basket in dutch oven, and sprinkle apples lightly with apple pie spice. Bring to a boil, cover tightly, and steam apples for 4–5 minutes or until crisp-tender. Remove from basket and place on a platter. Cool completely.

2. At serving time, spoon ½ teaspoon sauce over each apple half. Serve immediately.

SPICED CRANBERRY-POACHED PEARS

Serves 4

Total calories per serving: 99
Total fat per serving: 0.5 g (5%)

1½ cups low-calorie cranberry
    juice drink
¼ cup dry red wine
3 3-inch cinnamon sticks
8 whole cloves
3 medium-sized pears, peeled,
    quartered, and cored

1. In a dutch oven, combine cranberry juice, wine, cinnamon sticks, and cloves. Bring juice mixture to boil, add pear quarters, cover tightly, reduce heat, and simmer for 2 minutes. Turn pears and cook for 1½–2 minutes longer or until crisp-tender. Place three pear quarters in each of four individual dessert bowls or champagne glasses to cool.

2. Return juice mixture to a boil and boil for 2 minutes. Remove from heat and cool. Remove cinnamon sticks and cloves and pour equal amounts of sauce over pears. Chill for 1 hour.

CHOCOLATE-CRUMBLED BANANA CRESCENTS

Serves 4

Total calories per serving: 99
Total fat per serving: 2.8 g (25%)

2 medium-sized bananas
½ cup lite whipped topping
2 whole chocolate graham
    crackers, crumbled

Carefully slice bananas in half lengthwise and place one half cut side down on each of four individual dessert plates. Frost each banana half with 2 tablespoons whipped topping and sprinkle on one-fourth of cookie crumbs. Serve immediately or refrigerate.

SPARKLING GINGER FRUIT

Serves 4

Total calories per serving: 100
Total fat per serving: 0.8 g (7%)

14 medium-sized dark sweet
   cherries, halved and pitted
1 cup cantaloupe balls
1 cup seedless red or green grapes
1 cup honeydew balls
1 cup watermelon balls
1 cup fresh orange juice
1 cup sugar-free ginger ale
2 teaspoons grated orange zest

Arrange fruit in layers in a decorative glass bowl. In a small bowl, combine orange juice, ginger ale, and orange zest. Stir gently yet thoroughly to blend well. Pour over fruit and serve immediately.

FRUIT SMOOTHIES

Serves 4

Total calories per serving: 95
Total fat per serving: 0.2 g (2%)

1 16-ounce bag frozen mixed
   fruit
1 medium-sized banana
¾ cup vanilla nonfat yogurt

In a food processor, combine all ingredients and blend until smooth. Spoon into dessert bowls and serve immediately for a semisoft dessert or place in freezer for 30 minutes to freeze lightly. Stir gently and serve.

FROZEN TRIPLE COOKIES

Serves 4

Total calories per serving: 98
Total fat per serving: 2.7 g (25%)

¼ 3-ounce package sugar-free
   instant chocolate or vanilla
   pudding mix
½ cup skim milk
7 tablespoons lite whipped
   topping
12 thin chocolate wafers

1. In a mixing bowl, combine pudding mix and milk. Whisk until smooth. Chill for 20 minutes.

2. Gently but thoroughly fold in whipped topping. Spoon 1½ tablespoons of the pudding mixture onto each of four wafers, add another wafer on top of each, then add another 1½ tablespoons pudding and a third wafer. Wrap individually in plastic wrap and freeze.

Note: You may need to let the cookies stand for 4–5 minutes to soften before serving.

Variation: Add ¼ teaspoon peppermint extract to pudding mixture.

CREAMY STRAWBERRY ORANGE FROST

Serves 4

Total calories per serving: 98
Total fat per serving: 0.5 g (5%)

2 cups fresh orange juice
1⅓ cups frozen unsweetened
  whole strawberries
¼ cup nonfat dry milk
16 ice cubes
6 packets (2 teaspoons) Equal (if
  desired)
1 teaspoon vanilla extract
¼ teaspoon almond extract

In a food processor, combine all ingredients and blend until smooth. Pour into four chilled glasses and serve immediately.

CHOCOLATE FREEZER

Serves 4

Total calories per serving: 99
Total fat per serving: 0.1 g (1%)

½ teaspoon instant coffee
  granules
1 tablespoon hot water
1⅓ cups skim milk
16 ice cubes
1 teaspoon vanilla extract
1 tablespoon powdered sugar
4 packets (1⅓ teaspoons) Equal
1 cup chocolate nonfat frozen
  yogurt

Combine coffee granules and water and stir until completely dissolved. In a food processor, combine milk, ice cubes, vanilla, powdered sugar, sweetener, and coffee mixture; process until smooth. Add frozen yogurt and process until *just* blended. Pour into four glasses and serve with straws or pour into four wine goblets, place in freezer for 30 minutes, and serve with spoons.

COLOSSAL STRAWBERRY-ORANGE-GINGER COOLER

Serves 4

Total calories per serving: 97
Total fat per serving: 0.7 g (6%)

2⅔ cups fresh orange juice
2 cups frozen unsweetened
   strawberries
1 quart sugar-free ginger ale
Ice cubes

In a food processor, combine orange juice and frozen strawberries. Blend until smooth. Pour into four tall glasses and add 1 cup ginger ale to each. Stir gently yet thoroughly to blend. Fill with ice.

TROPICAL SNOW SLUSH

Serves 4

Total calories per serving: 91
Total fat per serving: 0.3 g (3%)

3 cups pineapple-orange juice or
   pineapple-orange-banana juice
1 cup sugar-free lemon-lime soda

Pour juice into ice trays and freeze overnight. Place one-fourth of the frozen cubes in a blender with ¼ cup soda at a time. Process until smooth and spoon into a chilled wineglass. Repeat with remaining ingredients. Serve with spoons.

MIXED FRUIT ICE POPS

Makes 12

Total calories per serving: 33
Total fat per serving: 0.2 g (5%)

2½ cups fresh or frozen
   unsweetened strawberries,
   thawed
1⅓ cups white grape juice
1 cup fresh orange juice

Place all ingredients in a blender and blend until smooth. Pour into 12 ⅓-cup ice pop molds and freeze.

SPICED APPLE AND CITRUS WARMER

Serves 4

Total calories per serving: 96
Total fat per serving: 0.2 g (2%)

1¾ cups unsweetened apple juice
1 cup unsweetened pineapple
   juice
1½ cups water
1 tablespoon sugar
1½ medium-sized lemons, peeled
   and sliced thin
1½ medium-sized oranges, peeled
   and sliced thin
2 3-inch cinnamon sticks
6 whole cloves

In a medium-sized saucepan, combine all ingredients, bring to a low simmer, and simmer, uncovered, for 15 minutes, occasionally stirring gently. Remove spices and serve.

HOT "BUTTERED" GROG

Serves 4

Total calories per serving: 100
Total fat per serving: 1 g (9%)

1 teaspoon ground cinnamon
¼ teaspoon ground nutmeg
⅛ teaspoon ground cloves
⅛ teaspoon ground allspice
1 teaspoon vanilla butternut
   flavoring
2 teaspoons light margarine
2 teaspoons sugar
2¾ cups apple juice
½ cup water
2 tablespoons dark rum
4 3-inch cinnamon sticks

1. In a small bowl, combine cinnamon, nutmeg, cloves, allspice, flavoring, margarine, and sugar. Using the back of a spoon, mash together until well blended. Chill until serving time.

2. In a medium-sized saucepan, combine apple juice, water, and rum. Bring to a boil and boil for 1 minute. Pour into four coffee mugs and stir in one-fourth of the spice mixture. Add cinnamon sticks and serve immediately.

INDEX